THE WHITEBOARD DAILY BOOK OF CUES

A VISUAL GUIDE TO EFFICIENT MOVEMENT FOR COACHES, TRAINERS, AND ATHLETES

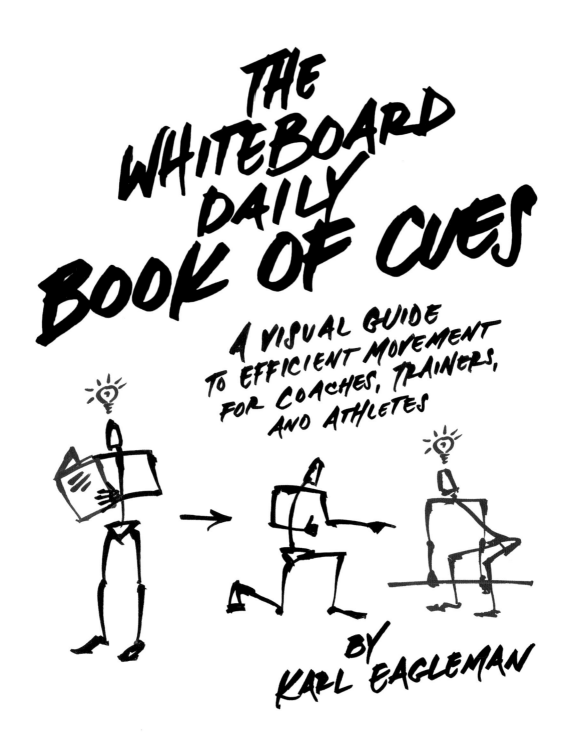

BY KARL EAGLEMAN

VICTORY BELT PUBLISHING INC.

LAS VEGAS

This book is dedicated to my daughter, Kadence. I hope it inspires you to discover and pursue your own unique passions.

First published in 2022 by Victory Belt Publishing Inc.

ISBN-13: 978-1-628601-45-9

Cover design by Karl Eagleman

Interior design by Kat Lannom

Illustrations by Karl Eagleman

Printed in Canada

TC 0222

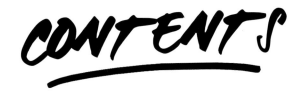

CONTENTS

INTRODUCTION | 4

CHAPTER 1: SQUAT | 8
AIR SQUAT | 9
BACK SQUAT | 20
FRONT SQUAT | 25
OVERHEAD SQUAT | 29
PISTOL SQUAT | 32
THERAPY | 34

CHAPTER 2: GYMNASTICS | 36
HANDSTAND | 37
HOLLOW ARCH POSITIONS | 40
JUMPING | 44
MUSCLE-UP | 45
PULL-UP | 59
PUSH-UP | 61
RING DIP | 67
SIT-UP | 69
T2B AND K2E | 70
WALL WALKS | 74

CHAPTER 3: DEADLIFT | 76

CHAPTER 4: OLY LIFTING | 102
JERK | 103
SNATCH & CLEAN | 127

CHAPTER 5: KETTLEBELL | 180

CHAPTER 6: RUNNING/
SPRINTING | 204

CHAPTER 7: ROWING | 212

CHAPTER 8: MOBILITY | 222

CHAPTER 9: BRACING | 230

CHAPTER 10: GRIP | 238

CHAPTER 11: POSITIONING | 256

CHAPTER 12: APPROACH | 262

CHAPTER 13: PERSPECTIVES | 282
EGO | 283
MINDSET | 294
MOVEMENT | 307
PACING | 312
PROGRESS | 319
RECOVERY | 334
RELATIONSHIPS | 340

CHAPTER 14: EDUCATION | 344
GENERAL | 345
ANATOMY | 352
TEACHING | 359
SEEING | 363
CORRECTING | 365
PRESENCE & ATTITUDE | 375
GROUP MANAGEMENT | 383
DEMONSTRATING | 387
PROGRAMMING | 389

ACKNOWLEDGMENTS | 394
FAN PHOTOS | 396
TITLE INDEX | 398

INTRODUCTION

In 2010, I distinctly remember being on the platform during an Olympic weightlifting session at Force Fitness in Bloomington, Indiana. Wil Fleming, my coach at the time, shared a cue with me to help me with my push jerk: "Down like a rock, up like a rocket." This mental visualization helped increase my understanding of the movement pattern and the explosive change of direction for the bar path. I thought, *Wouldn't it be cool if there was a massive "book of cues"—a giant comprehensive collection of cues—that could help both athletes and coaches communicate and understand movement?*

I kept this thought in the back of my mind for years, always hoping that I would someday get around to putting it together. However, I was always daunted by the size of the project. How in the world could someone create a massive list of coaching cues, and what would it look like?

In August 2017, I created the Instagram account @whiteboard_daily to share the significant amount of knowledge I'd gained throughout my years of being an athlete and coach.

At the time, I was in Ontario, Canada, traveling for work. During my travels, I sometimes carried a small square of whiteboard in my luggage. I used it to write up my workouts when exercising in hotel gyms, and my first post on @whiteboard_daily was the workout that I did in the parking lot of the hotel where I was staying.

At the time I made the first post, I didn't know exactly what I wanted WBD to be. I just knew I wanted to share my knowledge with others, and I felt like this account could be an outlet for me to do that.

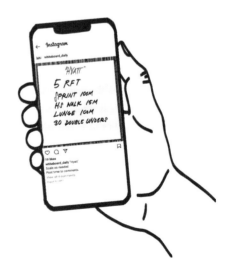

For the first few weeks, my content primarily consisted of workouts and motivational quotes, two things that are extremely common on social media. There was nothing special about this content, and the engagement on these posts was a clear indication of this. The posts garnered very few "likes" and comments.

However, I kept with it. Considering the name of the account was "Whiteboard Daily," I had locked myself into providing new content every twenty-four hours. After a couple months of posting workouts and quotes, I realized that there was nothing unique about what I was sharing. People who aren't family and friends of account owners follow accounts on social media for primarily two reasons: education or entertainment. WBD was really not providing much in either category.

I decided to map out a month of content ahead of time:

- **Monday:** Motivational quote
- **Tuesday:** Technique tip (coaching cue)
- **Wednesday:** Workout
- **Thursday:** Question for discussion in the comments
- **Friday:** Fitness tip
- **Saturday:** Coaching quote
- **Sunday:** Trivia

After sticking with this agenda for a few weeks, I quickly realized that the posts featuring coaching cues were by far the most engaging; they received more likes and comments compared to my other posts. Thankfully, these were the types of posts that I also enjoyed doing the most. Throughout my years of being an athlete and more than a decade of training CrossFit, I had mentally collected a small library of coaching cues that would be perfect to start sharing on WBD. From that point on, I began focusing the content that I posted on WBD to be more about coaching cues, and it has continued to grow from there.

More than anything, I created WBD because I simply wanted to help others get better at teaching and understanding movement. Now, that idea of creating a book to present the cues and education I've compiled over the years is coming to fruition!

HOW TO USE THIS BOOK AND THE CUES

In this book, the whiteboards are categorized as Coaching Cues, Skill Transfer, Movement Library, Coaching Education, and Coaching Perspective. The information on each whiteboard should be helpful regardless of whether you're a coach who's trying to help others or an athlete who's trying to improve on your own. And when it comes to the Coaching Education and Coaching Perspective tidbits, you may even find that they're applicable to your life outside of the gym.

Every good coach learns from other coaches, and by no means are all of the cues in this book my original ideas. You'll find a lot of hat tips (h/t) throughout the book, and I encourage you to check out the work of those coaches as well!

WHAT IS A CUE?

Cues are directions to improve movement. They give a body part a direction: "chest up," "knees out," "flex your butt." They should be specific, actionable, and short. This makes them easier to remember and quickly applicable.

Cues fall into four primary categories:

- **Verbal cues:** Using your voice to communicate movement—"JUMP!"
- **Visual cues:** Using your body to demonstrate movement—standing in front of your athlete and performing an air squat.
- **Mental cues:** Using imagery to describe movement—"Imagine you are screwing your feet into the ground."
- **Tactile cues:** Using touch or physical feedback to communicate what the athlete needs to do—squatting to a box.

A FEW THINGS TO CONSIDER

There is no such thing as a "golden cue." No cue works for every person every time. Since all athletes are unique and learn in different ways, it's important to have a variety of cues to address an issue. A larger mental toolbox gives you the potential to be an even better coach.

Give one cue at a time. When you watch a novice athlete move, they will likely display a number of movement inefficiencies. Rather than providing the athlete with a laundry list of items to fix, focus on the one that addresses their safety first and then triage from there. Hint: Work from the ground up when it comes to fixing movement. Most issues start with balance in the feet.

Cues should address the positive, not the negative. Saying, "Don't lower your elbows," doesn't provide specific instruction. The athlete may think, *Okay, then where* do *I put my elbows?* Tell the athlete what they *should do,* not the opposite.

Demonstrate the cue when you deliver it. Just as some people "talk with their hands," you should use your body to show what you mean when you say the cue.

Avoid using the same cue over and over again. If you do not see an improvement in the athlete's movement after you have provided a cue, try using a different cue or a combination of cues—e.g., tactile cue + verbal cue.

Know *when* to introduce a new cue. Warm-ups and working sets are the perfect time to deliver a new cue. This will be during a time when the athlete is fresh and the weight is manageable. Never introduce a new cue when the athlete is attempting to lift a weight that is more than 80 percent of their one-rep max (1RM). During that time, it is important for the athlete to focus on familiar concepts that have proven to work for them.

Get creative! Maya Angelou said, "You can't use up creativity. The more you use, the more you have." The same applies to communicating movement. The exercises we do in the gym are supposed to make us stronger for our activity in the real world. Use that connection to make movement relatable.

ONE LAST THING

I sincerely hope this book brings you value. Again, my mission is to help coaches, athletes, and anyone who wants to improve their own movement. Take what you have learned from this book and use it to help other people. Use these cues with your athletes. Mash them up. Remix them. Put your own spin on them. Make them better! Most importantly, have fun—and find some time to draw on a whiteboard.

CHAPTER ①

SQUAT

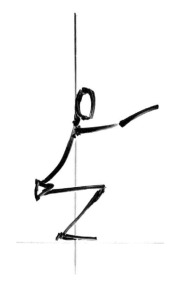

AIR SQUAT

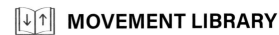

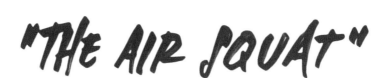

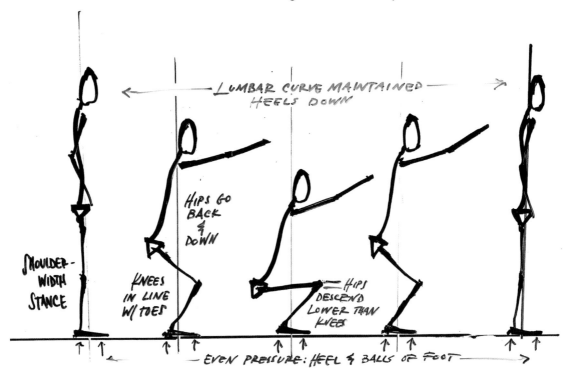

Points of performance

- The feet should be in a shoulder-width stance.

- The hips descend back and down and go lower than the knees.

- The lumbar curve is maintained.

- The heels stay grounded.

- The knee direction is in line with the toe direction.

- The movement is complete at full hip and knee extension.

COACHING CUE

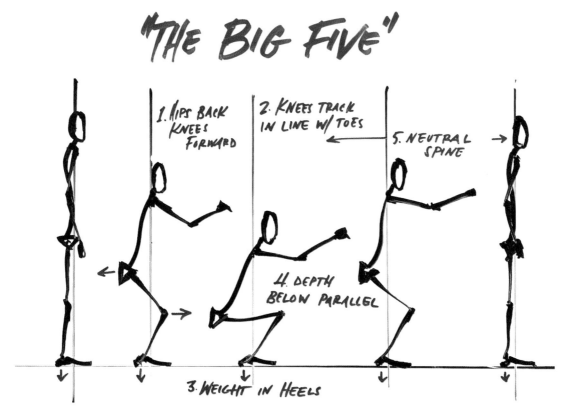

h/t Denise Thomas (@denthomas7)

What does this mean?

The Big Five refers to the five points of performance coaches use to evaluate and assess the mechanics of the air squat:

1. The hips are back, and the knees are forward.
2. The knees track in-line with the toes.
3. The weight is in the heels.
4. Depth goes below parallel.
5. Neutral spine is maintained.

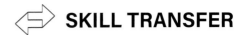
SQUATTING → SITTING ON THE TOILET

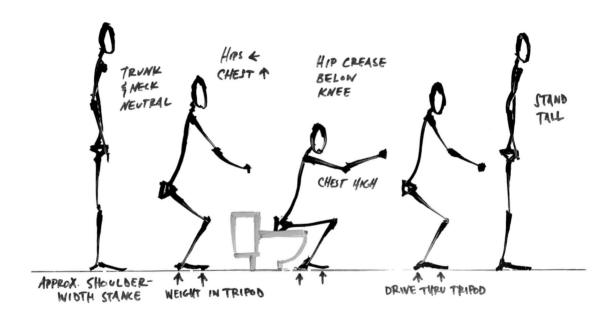

What does this mean?

When considering a hierarchy of functional movements, there are few exercises more transferable from the gym to real-life situations than the squat.

If you will be sitting down on and standing up from a toilet, you can be sure that the squat should be a part of your normal exercise routine.

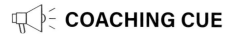

GROCERY BAG / CAR DOOR

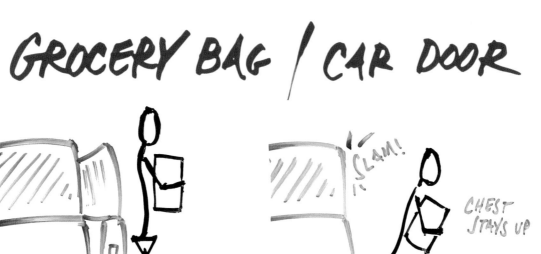

When

This cue can be used to teach the athlete to lead into the squat by sending their hips back while keeping the chest up.

Why is this cue important?

- **Hips initially go back:** Before descending, the hips and knees must unlock.

- **Chest stays up:** Keeping the chest up helps the athlete maintain a lumbar curve.

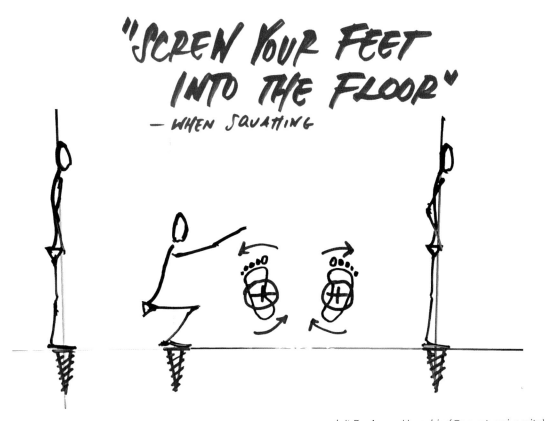

h/t Dr. Aaron Horschig (@squat_university)

When?

Use this cue for any type of squat (air, back, front, etc.).

What does this mean?

When squatting, the idea is to recruit as many of the right muscles as possible. It is important to make the connection between the mind and body. Telling the athlete to "screw your feet into the floor" helps accomplish both of these.

The athlete should imagine having screws extending from their feet into the ground. Then they initiate a rotation from their hips, through their legs, and into the ground through their feet (the "righty-tighty" rule does not apply here). They jam their toes and heels into the ground so their feet do not slide. When the athlete correctly grips the ground with their feet, they set a firm foundation to perform a strong squat.

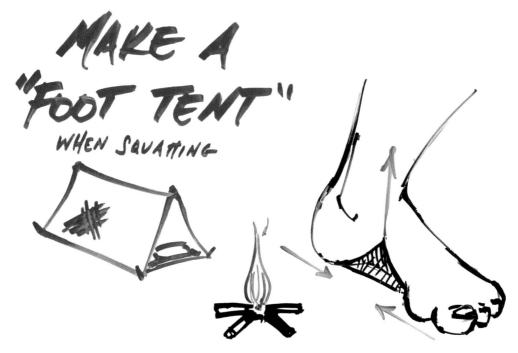

MAKE A "FOOT TENT" WHEN SQUATTING

h/t Dr. Katie Clare (@drkatie_clare)

What does this mean?

Often an issue with the knees or hips is caused from having little to no engagement from the muscles in the foot.

Making a foot tent means activating the muscles in the foot to pull the arch high and jam the toes down. The foot is packed with muscles. Use them!

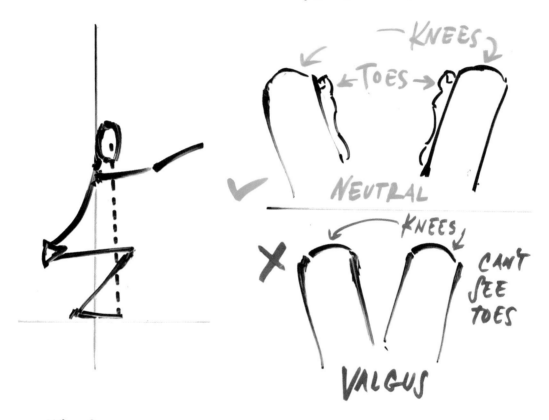

"SEE YOUR BIG TOE"
DURING THE SQUAT

When?
Use this cue to ensure the athlete's knees track over the toes during the air squat.

What does this mean?
Throughout the squat movement, if the athlete looks down from a neutral head position, they should be able to see their big toes. This indicates the knees are tracking correctly. The knees blocking the athlete's line of sight to the big toe indicates knee valgus (knees caving in).

📢 COACHING CUE

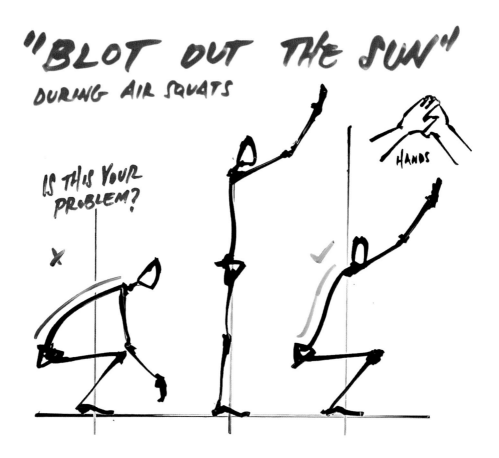

"BLOT OUT THE SUN"
DURING AIR SQUATS

IS THIS YOUR PROBLEM?

HANDS

When?

Use this cue to help an athlete who tends to bow forward when they squat.

What does this mean?

The athlete should stand tall and extend their arms slightly above their head (~45°), as if they are "blotting out the sun" and creating shade. Then they keep their arms in this position as they move through the full range of movement of their squat.

Why?

Loss of a neutral spine in a squat puts the athlete in a weak, compromised position. Extending their arms above their head helps keep their chest up and activates muscles in their back, leading to better positioning.

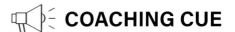
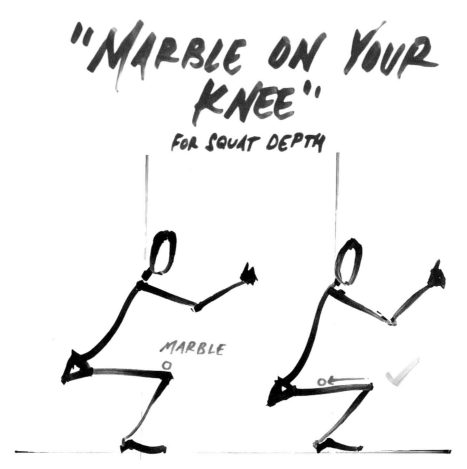

"MARBLE ON YOUR KNEE"

FOR SQUAT DEPTH

MARBLE

h/t Meg Ridley (@meggiesue19)

When?

Use this cue to establish hip crease below the knee in the squat.

What does this mean?

At the bottom of the squat, cue the athlete to pause and imagine a marble is on their knee. If the imaginary marble would roll toward their hip, the hip crease is below the knee.

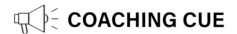

COACHING CUE

"SHOW ME YOUR SHIRT"

WHENEVER CUEING "CHEST UP"

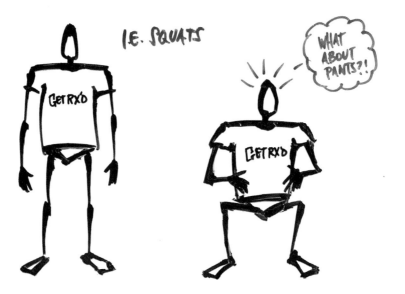

IE. SQUATS

When?

Use this cue to remind the athlete to keep their chest up during squats, deadlifts, etc.

What does this mean?

By cueing the athlete to keep their posture upright so that you can see the front of their shirt, you may prevent them from bowing forward during their lifts.

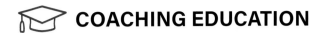
"THE SQUAT IS ESSENTIAL TO YOUR WELL-BEING."
— GREG GLASSMAN

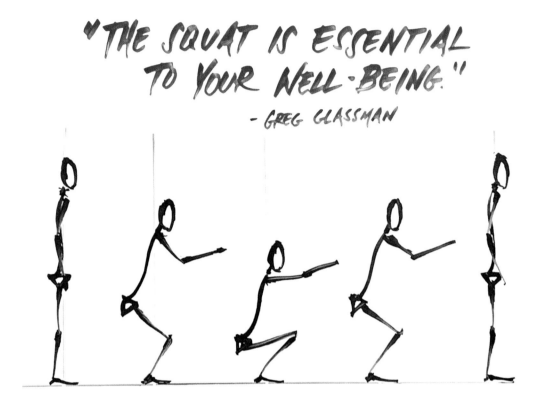

What does this mean?

Few exercises done in a gym setting carry more transferability to real life than the squat. (The deadlift places a close second.) Sitting down and standing up is as big a part of a normal routine as any other activity. Athletes who strengthen the biomechanics of this movement improve the quality of their well-being.

BACK SQUAT

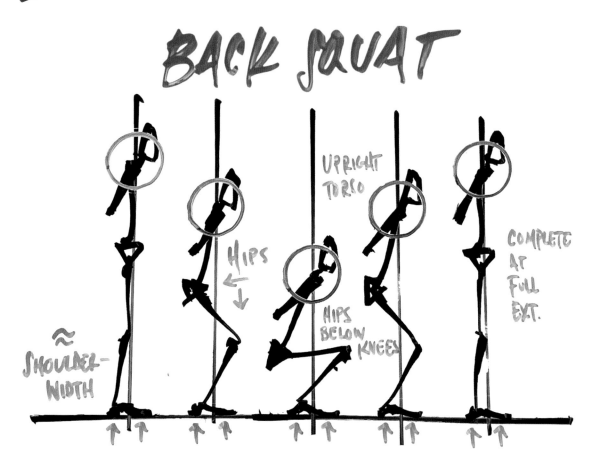

BACK SQUAT

≈ SHOULDER-WIDTH

HIPS

UPRIGHT TORSO

HIPS BELOW KNEES

COMPLETE AT FULL EXT.

Points of performance

- The feet should be in a shoulder-width stance.
- The hands should be just outside the shoulders with a full grip on the bar.
- The bar rests on the upper back.
- The hips descend back and down and go lower than the knees.
- The lumbar curve is maintained.
- The heels stay grounded.
- The knee direction is in line with the toe direction.
- The movement is complete at full hip and knee extension.

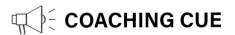
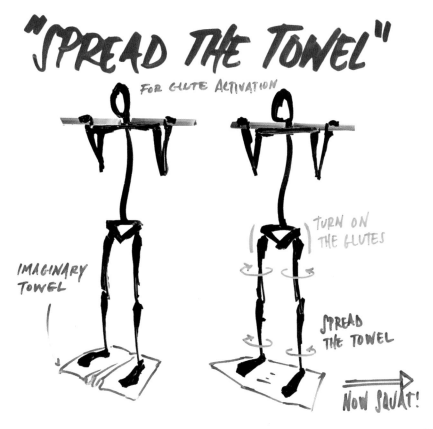

"SPREAD THE TOWEL"

FOR GLUTE ACTIVATION

IMAGINARY TOWEL

TURN ON THE GLUTES

SPREAD THE TOWEL

NOW SQUAT!

Picked up from Eugen Loki (@pheasyque)

When?

Use this cue to describe how to create lower body tension.

What does this mean?

Similar to "Screw Your Feet into the Floor," this cue may help your athlete further understand how to engage the musculature in the lower body, especially during a squat.

The athlete should pretend they have a crumpled towel under their feet. They spread the towel out by screwing their feet to the floor, which engages the glutes to create tension in the lower body before they start the squat eccentric.

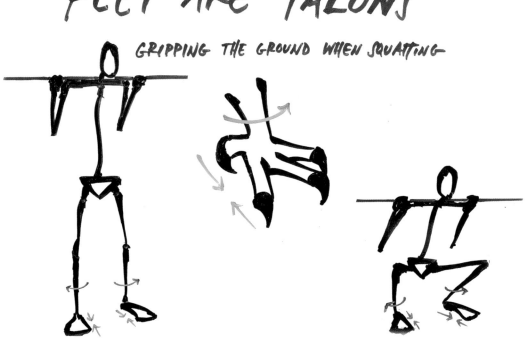

"FEET ARE TALONS"
GRIPPING THE GROUND WHEN SQUATTING

h/t Jason Ackerman (@coachjasonackerman)

What does this mean?

The athlete statically activates the foot muscles to maintain the arch similar to the squeeze of a hawk's talons.

Why?

A stable base starts from the ground up to balance the load on all joints and bones.

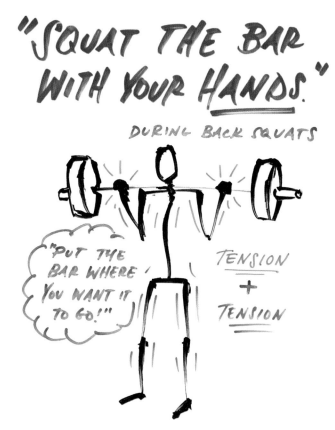

h/t Lee Boyce (@coachleeboyce)

What does this mean?

Tension has to come from both the upper and lower halves of the athlete's body. Actively pulling apart on the bar creates tension through the entire back and also takes some of the pressure of the bar off your back.

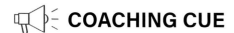
COACHING CUE

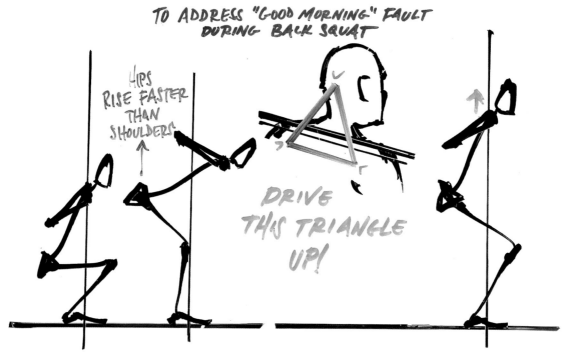

h/t Donnie "SuperD" Thompson (@thompsonbowtie)

When?

Use this cue to fix the "good morning" fault.

What does this mean?

The "good morning" fault occurs when the hips rise out of the bottom of the squat faster than the shoulders. This places the athlete in a compromised position and changes the movement pattern from a squat to a "good morning."

To address this issue, cue the athlete to visualize a triangle that is on the upper traps and the back of the head. The athlete needs to "drive the triangle straight up."

FRONT SQUAT

THE FRONT SQUAT

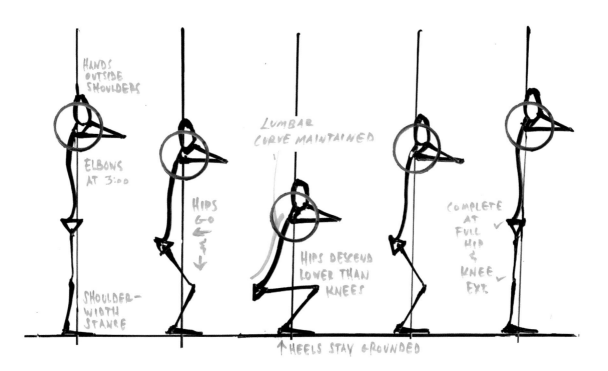

Points of performance

- The feet should be in a shoulder-width stance.
- The hands should be just outside of the shoulders.
- The grip on the bar is loose, with just the fingertips.
- The elbows are high.
- The hips descend back and down and go lower than the knees.
- The lumbar curve is maintained.
- The heels stay grounded.
- The knees are in line with the toes.
- The movement is complete at full hip and knee extension.

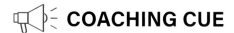
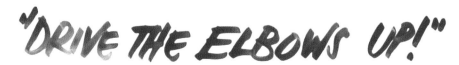

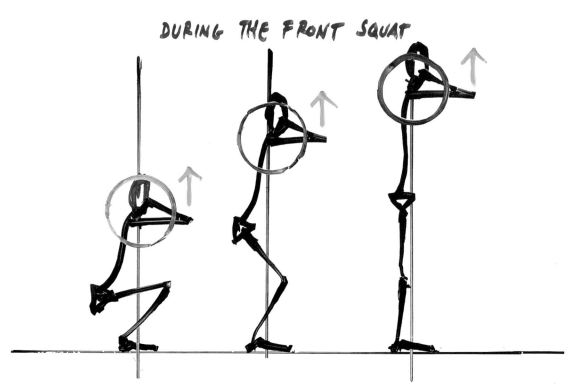

Why?

Driving the elbows high throughout the front squat, especially when standing up, places the athlete in a stronger position by keeping the bar close to the midline of the body and the torso stacked upright.

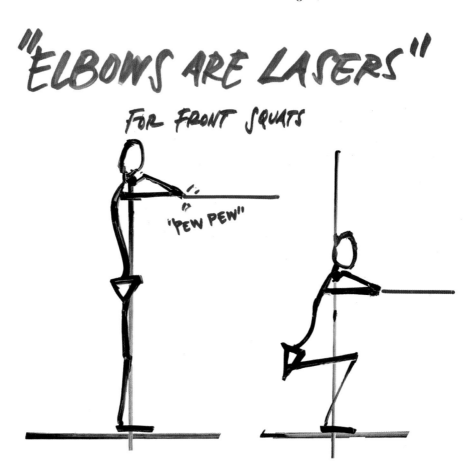

"ELBOWS ARE LASERS"
FOR FRONT SQUATS

"PEW PEW"

What does this mean?

Cue an athlete who's holding the bar in the front-rack position to point their elbows straight forward, as if they are shooting lasers directly ahead. Instruct them to keep that elbow position throughout the full range of the squat.

Why?

When done correctly, this will create a shelf for the bar to sit comfortably on top of the shoulders and chest. Additionally, this position will help keep the weight of the bar as close to the midline as possible.

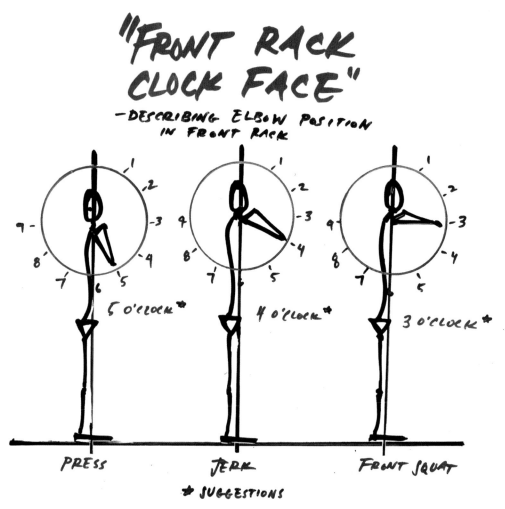

"FRONT RACK CLOCK FACE"
— DESCRIBING ELBOW POSITION IN FRONT RACK

PRESS — 5 o'clock*

JERK — 4 o'clock*

FRONT SQUAT — 3 o'clock*

* SUGGESTIONS

h/t Oleksiy Torokhtiy (@torokhtiy)

When?

Use this cue to help the athlete position their elbows correctly in the front rack based on the type of lift they're doing.

What does this mean?

Referencing the hours on a clock to describe the position of the elbows may help the athlete visualize their position correctly. For example:

- **Press:** Elbows at 5 o'clock position
- **Jerk:** Elbows at 4 o'clock position
- **Front squat:** Elbows at 3 o'clock position

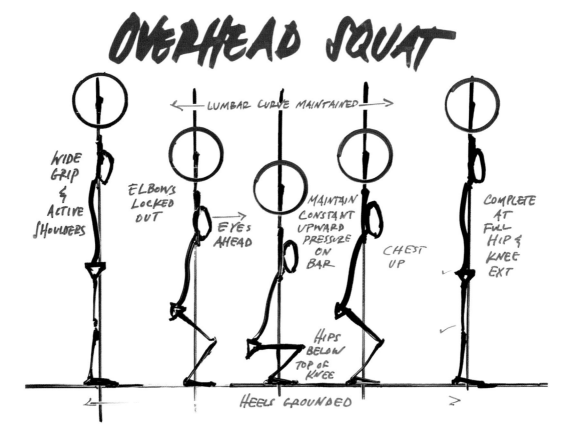

OVERHEAD SQUAT

LUMBAR CURVE MAINTAINED

WIDE GRIP & ACTIVE SHOULDERS

ELBOWS LOCKED OUT

EYES AHEAD

MAINTAIN CONSTANT UPWARD PRESSURE ON BAR

CHEST UP

COMPLETE AT FULL HIP & KNEE EXT

HIPS BELOW TOP OF KNEE

HEELS GROUNDED

Points of performance

- The athlete should be in a stance that allows a full range of motion below parallel.

- The athlete uses a wide grip on the bar.

- The shoulders are active (elbows pointed down, armpits pointing forward).

- The elbows are locked out.

- The trunk and neck remain in a neutral position.

- While overhead, the bar stays aligned over the middle of the foot.

- The weight stays in the tripod of the foot (see page 38).

- The chest stays high.

- The knees are in line with the toes.

- The athlete reaches the full range of motion (below parallel).

- The movement is complete at full knee and hip extension with the bar aligned over the center of the foot.

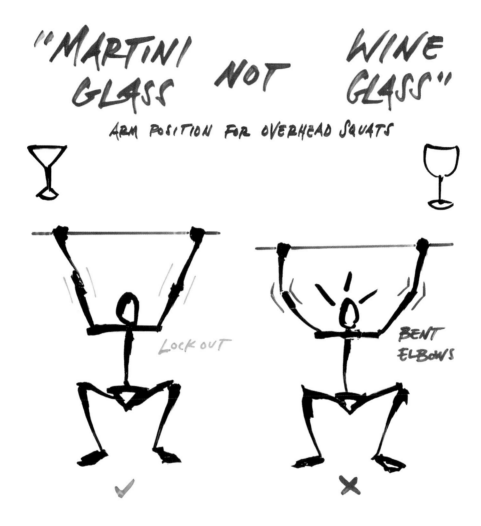

When?

Use this cue to remind the athlete of proper arm position during the overhead squat.

What does this mean?

The arm position should mimic the straight sides of a martini glass, not the curved sides of a wine glass.

Why?

To keep the barbell overhead in a firm position, the athlete's elbows should be completely locked out.

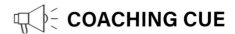
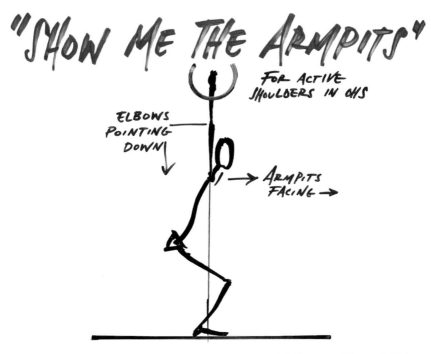

h/t Burgener Strength (@burgenerstrength)

When?

Use this cue to remind the athlete to activate their shoulders while in the overhead squat position.

What does this mean?

The athlete should point their armpits forward and their elbows down to the floor. As with all barbell cues, the athlete should work through this cue while using a PVC pipe and revisit it while working with a bar and adding weight.

Why?

Pointing the armpits forward and the elbows down creates external rotation and activates muscles in the back, including the large latissimus dorsi.

> *"It's the only position you can be in to handle heavy weight over your head."*

—Mike Burgener

PISTOL SQUAT

THE PISTOL

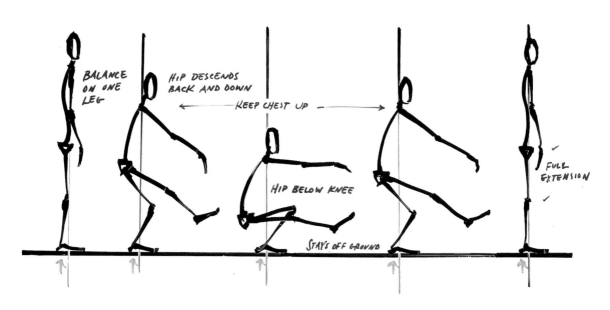

BALANCE ON ONE LEG

HIP DESCENDS BACK AND DOWN

← KEEP CHEST UP →

HIP BELOW KNEE

STAYS OFF GROUND

FULL EXTENSION

Points of performance

- Balance on one leg, with the nonworking leg in front of the body.

- The hip for the standing leg descends back and down and goes lower than the knee.

- The knee of the standing leg stays in line with the toes, and the heel stays down.

- The nonworking leg does not touch the ground.

- The move is complete at full hip and knee extension of the standing leg.

- The chest stays up as much as possible.

Need more help?

Check out "Pistol Squat Jackpot Program" from @performanceplusprogram with @pamelagnon.

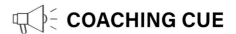
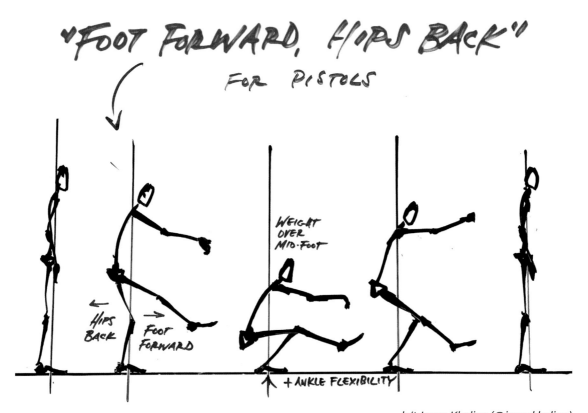

"FOOT FORWARD, HIPS BACK"
FOR PISTOLS

HIPS BACK

FOOT FORWARD

WEIGHT OVER MID-FOOT

+ ANKLE FLEXIBILITY

h/t Jason Khalipa (@jasonkhalipa)

What does this mean?

The pistol requires a fair amount of balance in addition to flexibility and strength. Pushing the lead foot forward and pulling the hips back will help keep the athlete's bodyweight over the supporting foot.

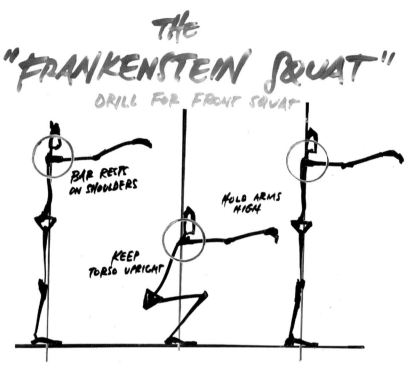

THE "FRANKENSTEIN SQUAT" DRILL FOR FRONT SQUAT

BAR RESTS ON SHOULDERS

HOLD ARMS HIGH

KEEP TORSO UPRIGHT

When?

This movement is a great drill to help the athlete understand the position of the bar during the front squat.

Points of performance

- The feet are in a shoulder-width stance.

- The feet are slightly turned out.

- The bar is securely in the channel between the top of the shoulders and base of the throat.

- The arms are extended in front of the body.

- The arms are held high, and the shoulders are square to prevent the bar from rolling forward.

- The hips descend back and down and go lower than the knees.

- The lumbar curve is maintained.

- The heels stay grounded.

- The knees are in line with the toes.

- The move is complete at full hip and knee extension.

CHAPTER ②

GYMNASTICS

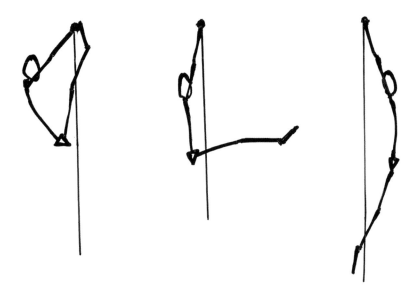

HANDSTAND

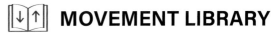
HANDSTAND PUSH-UP

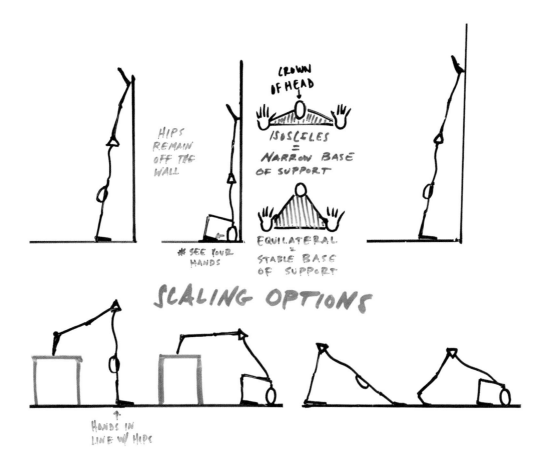

Points of performance

- The hands are positioned just outside shoulder width.
- The arms are extended.
- The elbows move forward so the head descends until it touches the ground.
- The abdominals remain braced.
- The move is complete at full arm extension with a straight line of the body.

THE TRIPOD

CROWN OF HEAD

X NARROW BASE OF SUPPORT
X FINGERS OUT OF PERIPHERAL
X NARROW FINGER POSITION

CROWN OF HEAD

THINK
EQUILATERAL
TRIANGLE
NOT
ISOSCELES
TRIANGLE.

✔ WIDE BASE OF SUPPORT
✔ FINGERS IN PERIPHERAL
✔ WIDE FLAT HANDS

When?

Athletes looking to get upside down must learn to be comfortable in the tripod or headstand. The most common flaw I see with my athletes is the base of support is far too narrow.

Points of performance

- Broad base of support (equilateral triangle rather than isosceles). This is easy to see when using a mat. The top of the head and hand positions will leave a mark (usually sweat and chalk), so the athlete can see where their positioning was when they were inverted.

- Fingers should be visible in the athlete's peripheral vision.

- Hands should be wide and flat.

Why?

An unstable position is a weak position. These cues may help athletes gain stability in this movement.

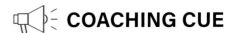
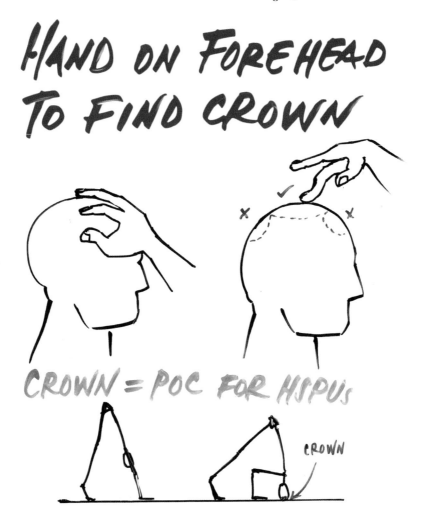

HAND ON FOREHEAD TO FIND CROWN

CROWN = POC FOR HSPUs

CROWN

When?

When coaching, you could simply say "top of your head," but, believe it or not, this is a relative location, especially with novice movers. Instead, offer the "hand on forehead" cue to athletes to identify the crown of the head, especially during headstands and handstand push-ups. This self-tactile cue will allow your athlete to quickly and accurately identify exactly where the crown of their head is located.

Why?

This specific point of contact with the floor is imperative because any deviation can place the head and neck in a compromised and weak position.

BE A "LEAF SPRING"
FOR HOLLOW POSITION

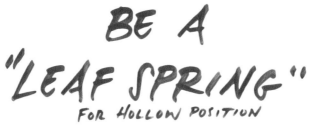

TENSION · EXTENSION · TENSION

"LOW BACK" ON FLOOR

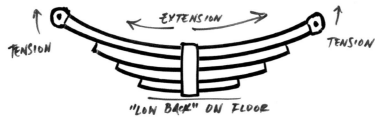

ARMS BY EARS · POSTERIOR TILT · KNEES & ELBOWS EXTENDED · POINTED TOES

LOW BACK TOUCHING GROUND

What does this mean?

A leaf spring is a slender arc-shaped length of spring steel. This shape and the tension it provides is similar to that of the hollow body position.

Points of performance

- No space between the lumbar spine and the floor.

- The scapulae are elevated off the ground.

- The hips are extended with a posterior pelvic tilt.

- The knees and elbows are locked.

- The arms are by the ears with active shoulders.

- The ankles are in plantar flexion with pointed toes.

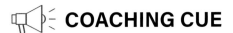
"RIB CAGE TO PELVIS"

FOR HOLLOW BODY

NEUTRAL

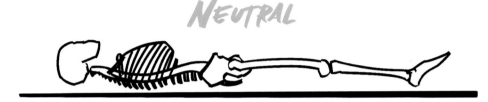

HOLLOW

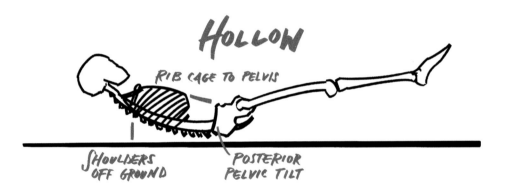

RIB CAGE TO PELVIS

SHOULDERS OFF GROUND

POSTERIOR PELVIC TILT

What does this mean?

The athlete should flex their abdominal muscles, round their back, and bring the points of their rib cage toward their pelvis.

COACHING CUE

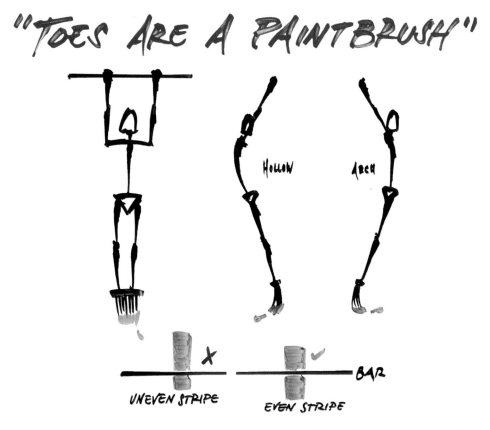

"TOES ARE A PAINTBRUSH"

h/t Chuck Bennington (@chuckbennington)

When?

Use this cue as a kipping drill or warm-up. The athlete hangs from the bar, transitioning through hollow to arch positions.

What does this mean?

The athlete can imagine that their toes are a paintbrush as they hang from the bar. As they transition through the hollow and arch positions, they paint a line on the floor that extends an equal distance on either side.

Why?

This drill helps the athlete do the following:

- Build control and body awareness
- Understand the feeling of being even under the bar
- Keep their legs zipped together and toes pointed

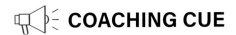

"SPINE ABOVE SHOULDER BLADES"

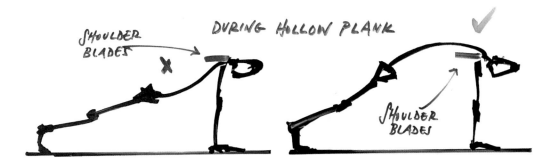

When?

Use this cue for establishing the hollow body position during a plank.

What does this mean?

When the athlete is in the plank position, cue them to push away from the ground so their spine is higher than their shoulder blades. Other similar cues are

- "Spine to ceiling"
- "Push the earth away"
- "Get punched in the chest"

Why?

This small adjustment will help the athlete engage the muscles throughout their core to establish a hollow body position.

JUMPING

"STANDING BROAD JUMP"

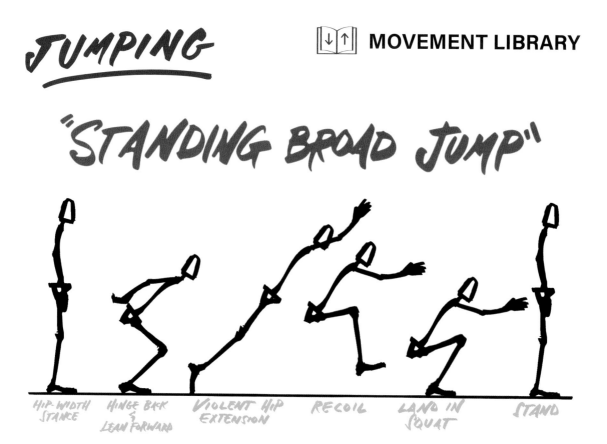

HIP-WIDTH STANCE · HINGE BACK & LEAN FORWARD · VIOLENT HIP EXTENSION · RECOIL · LAND IN SQUAT · STAND

Points of performance

- The feet are in a hip-width stance.
- The athlete hinges the hips back and leans forward with the arms behind the body.
- The arms swing forward as the athlete rapidly extends the hips and knees.
- The athlete recoils and lands in a squat.
- The movement is complete when the athlete stands to full extension.

MUSCLE-UP

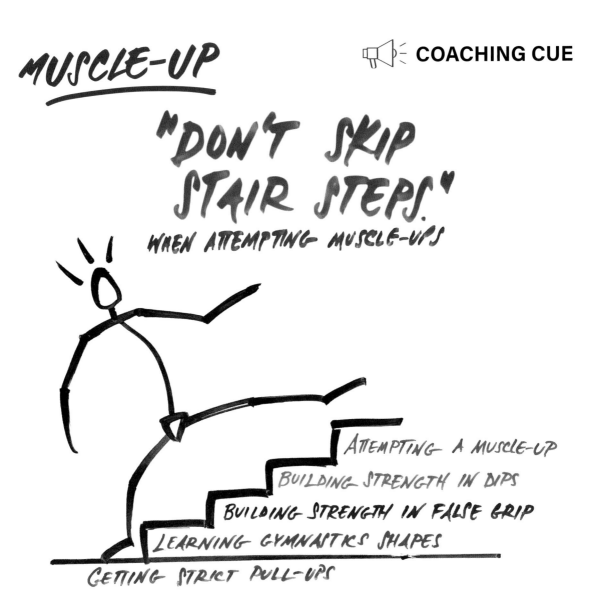

"DON'T SKIP STAIR STEPS."
WHEN ATTEMPTING MUSCLE-UPS

ATTEMPTING A MUSCLE-UP
BUILDING STRENGTH IN DIPS
BUILDING STRENGTH IN FALSE GRIP
LEARNING GYMNASTICS SHAPES
GETTING STRICT PULL-UPS

What does this mean?

It's no surprise the siren song of the muscle-up lures even the least-skilled athletes with its symphony of human motion. However, as movements build in complexity, they also require a broader and deeper range of preparation. This illustration may help you communicate to your athlete the steps required before attempting a muscle-up.

"BAD CHEERLEADER JUMP"

FOR BAR MUSCLE-UP APPROACH

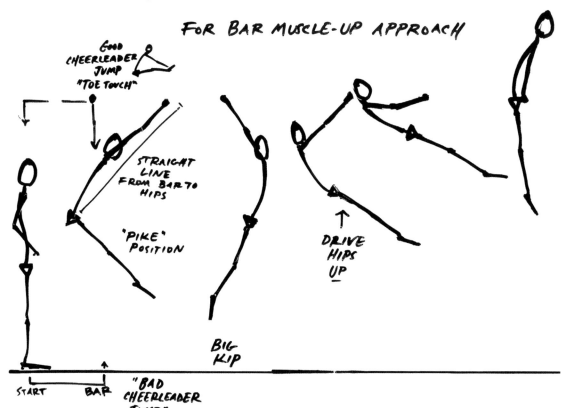

GOOD CHEERLEADER JUMP "TOE TOUCH"

STRAIGHT LINE FROM BAR TO HIPS

"PIKE" POSITION

DRIVE HIPS UP

BIG KIP

START   BAR   "BAD CHEERLEADER JUMP"

Travis Ewart (@travis_ewart, @invictus_gymnastics)

When?

Use this cue to help the athlete as they're approaching the bar for a bar muscle-up.

What does this mean?

The "bad cheerleader jump" is essentially a jump in the pike position toward the bar. When done correctly, the jump may provide the athlete with the added momentum needed to drive their hips toward the bar to complete a bar muscle-up.

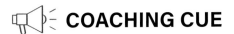
"FALL INTO PIKE"

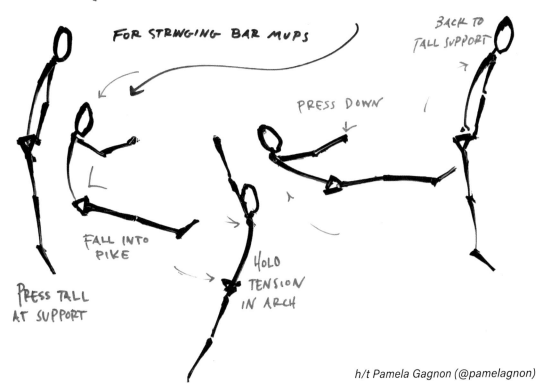

FOR STRINGING BAR MUPS

BACK TO TALL SUPPORT

PRESS DOWN

FALL INTO PIKE

HOLD TENSION IN ARCH

PRESS TALL AT SUPPORT

h/t Pamela Gagnon (@pamelagnon)

When?

Use this cue to help an athlete who is working on stringing together bar muscle-ups.

What does this mean?

- The athlete should stay tight as they fall back into a pike.
- They should hold tension in the arch.
- They should press down and around.
- They should press *tall* at the top into support.

Need more help?

For more information on all things gymnastics, I highly suggest you follow @pamelagnon on Instagram.

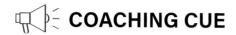
COACHING CUE

"FEET IN A BUCKET"

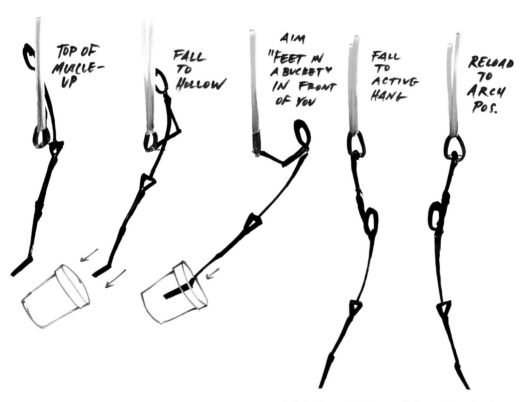

TOP OF MUSCLE-UP

FALL TO HOLLOW

AIM "FEET IN A BUCKET" IN FRONT OF YOU

FALL TO ACTIVE HANG

RELOAD TO ARCH POS.

h/t Andrew Charlesworth (@andrewcharlesworth1)

When?

Use this cue for athletes who are working on cycling ring muscle-ups.

What does this mean?

On the descent from the support position during a muscle-up, the athlete should try to put their feet in an imaginary bucket in front of them. Doing so prevents their legs from dissipating the kip so they can gain the most momentum.

"HIGH INSIDE PITCH"

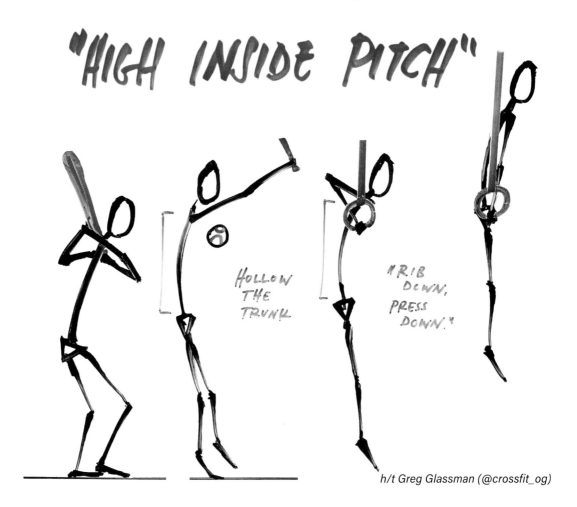

HOLLOW THE TRUNK

"RIB DOWN, PRESS DOWN."

h/t Greg Glassman (@crossfit_og)

When?

Use this cue when coaching an athlete to roll over the rings in the muscle-up transition.

What does this mean?

The muscle-up involves a strong ab contraction that "hollows" the trunk, which makes rolling over the rings much easier. The motion may remind the athlete of dodging a "high-inside" pitch.

"KIPPING RING MUSCLE-UP"

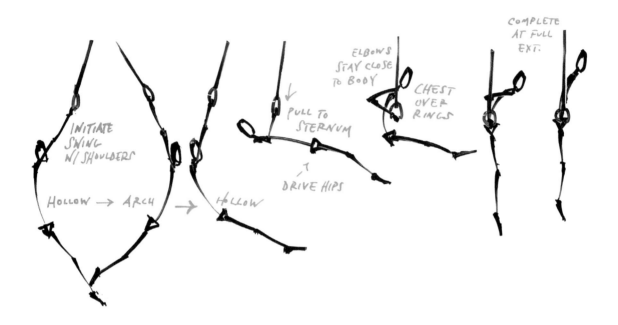

COMPLETE AT FULL EXT.

ELBOWS STAY CLOSE TO BODY

CHEST OVER RINGS

PULL TO STERNUM

INITIATE SWING N/ SHOULDERS

DRIVE HIPS

HOLLOW → ARCH → HOLLOW

Points of performance

- The rings should be set approximately shoulder width apart.

- The athlete should use a false grip or regular grip on the rings.

- The athlete should start in a hanging position with arms extended.

- The athlete initiates the swing with the shoulders.

- The movement alternates between hollow and arch positions.

- The athlete drives the hips toward the rings while in the hollow position.

- The athlete pulls the rings to the sternum as the torso leans back.

- The chest moves over the rings while the hands and elbows stay close to the body.

- The movement is complete at full arm extension in the support position.

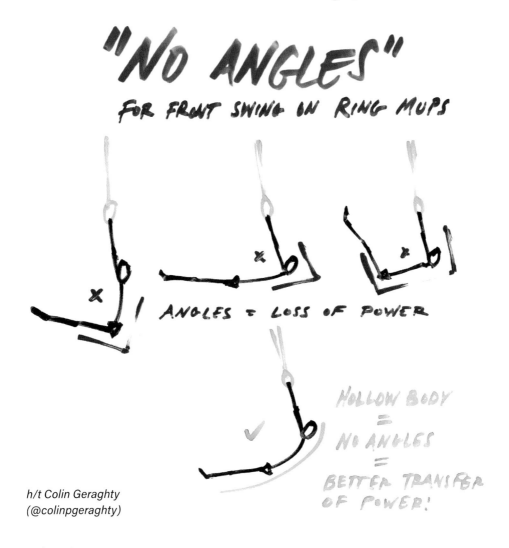

"NO ANGLES"
FOR FRONT SWING ON RING MUPS

ANGLES = LOSS OF POWER

HOLLOW BODY
=
NO ANGLES
=
BETTER TRANSFER OF POWER!

*h/t Colin Geraghty
(@colinpgeraghty)*

When?

This cue is intended to help athletes during the front swing on ring muscle-ups.

What does this mean?

You may have heard the cue, "When the arms bend, the power ends," applied to Olympic weightlifting (credit to @mikeburgener). The same can be said in regard to ring muscle-ups.

When angles are created on the front swing of the ring muscle-up (through the hips, shoulders, or both), there is a loss of power transfer. However, no angles = hollow body = efficient transfer of power.

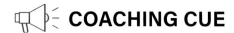

ONLY TWO SHAPES

DURING A KIPPING MUSCLE-UP

TIGHT ARCH **AND HOLLOW BODY**

h/t CrossFit Gymnastics (@thegymnasticscourse)

When?

This cue applies to kipping muscle-ups.

What does this mean?

In an efficient rep of a kipping muscle-up, the body should create only two shapes: the hollow and the arch. Any extra angle created is technically more work.

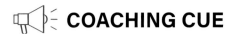
"RIB DOWN. PRESS DOWN"

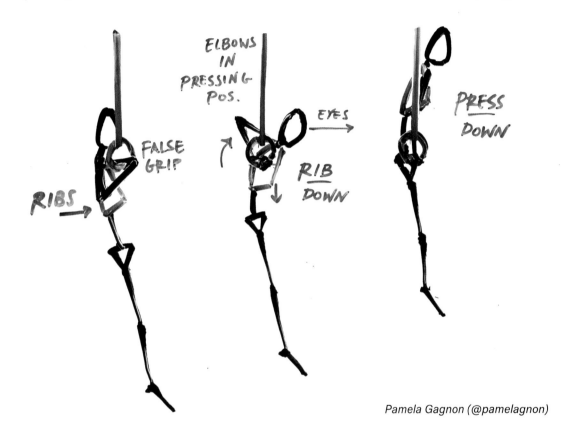

ELBOWS IN PRESSING POS.

EYES

FALSE GRIP

RIBS

RIB DOWN

PRESS DOWN

Pamela Gagnon (@pamelagnon)

When?

This cue applies to athletes doing toes to bar but can also apply to ring muscle-ups.

What does this mean?

The distance for the toes to travel to the bar can be made much shorter by employing the hollow compression on the back swing.

> *"Practice pulling 'rib down, press down' as opposed to 'rib out, arch behind.'"*
>
> —@pamelagnon

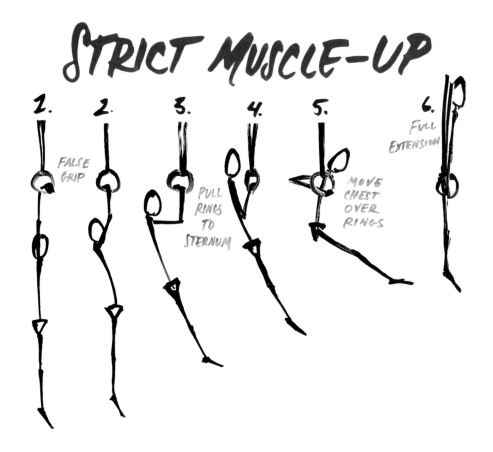

STRICT MUSCLE-UP

1. FALSE GRIP

2.

3. PULL RINGS TO STERNUM

4.

5. MOVE CHEST OVER RINGS

6. FULL EXTENSION

Points of performance

- The rings should be set approximately shoulder width apart.

- The rings are held in a false grip.

- The athlete starts by hanging with the arms extended.

- The athlete pulls the rings to the sternum as the torso leans back.

- The chest moves over the rings while the hands and elbows stay close to the body.

- The movement is complete at the support position with full arm extension.

Why?

Focusing on performing a strict muscle-up before doing a kipping muscle-up helps athletes build the upper body strength to handle the dynamic movement of the kipping swing.

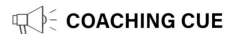
"THUMBS TRACE YOUR CHEST"

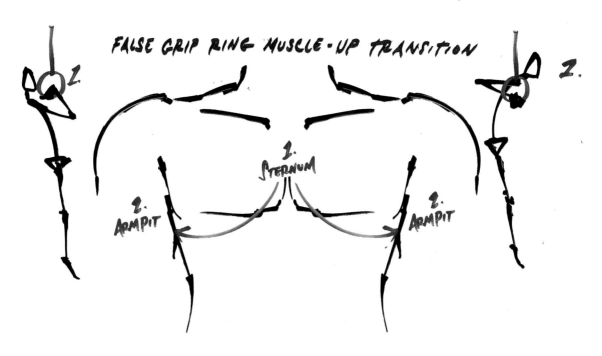

FALSE GRIP RING MUSCLE-UP TRANSITION

1. STERNUM

2. ARMPIT

2. ARMPIT

When?

Use this cue for teaching the transition for the false grip ring muscle-up.

What does this mean?

The transition of the muscle-up occurs when the shoulders move from below the rings to above the rings. During the transition of the false grip ring muscle-up, the athlete should pull the rings so the knuckles of the hands face each other. They pull the rings to the chest, and then the thumbs trace the chest from sternum to armpit. Doing so will position the shoulders above the rings so the athlete is ready to press into the support position.

📣 COACHING CUE

"IT'S MUSCLE-UP, NOT MUSCLE-FORWARD"

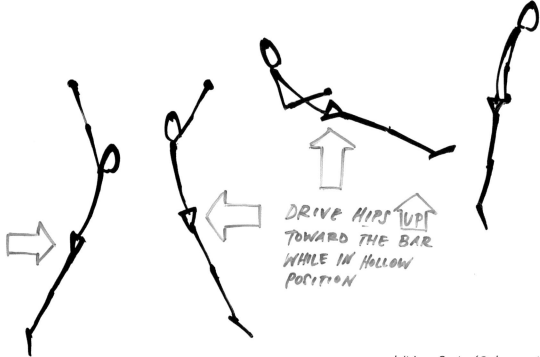

DRIVE HIPS UP
TOWARD THE BAR
WHILE IN HOLLOW
POSITION

h/t Juan Castro (@cjuan.castro, CrossFit Gymnastics lead coach)

When?

Use this cue to coach both bar muscle-ups and ring muscle-ups.

What does this mean?

Gravity is already working against the athlete. If they drop their chest through/forward, their body will follow and make things more difficult. If the athlete pulls to land "tall," their dip will be much easier.

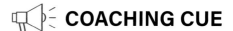

"TOWEL BETWEEN THE FEET"

DURING HOLLOW & ARCH POSITIONS

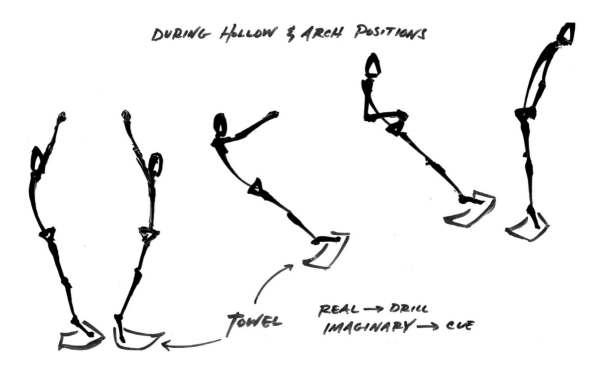

TOWEL

REAL → DRILL
IMAGINARY → CUE

When?

Use this cue when the athlete is working in hollow and tight arch positions, such as hanging, support, rocks, and handstands. This cue also can be used as a drill.

What does this mean?

The athlete should zip the legs together and point the feet to activate muscles throughout the entire lower body. Whether the athlete imagines holding a towel between the feet or actually does so, this cue/drill helps the athlete keep the legs together and toes pointed.

Why?

When the body works together as a single lever, more efficient power is produced.

THE "PULL-OVER"

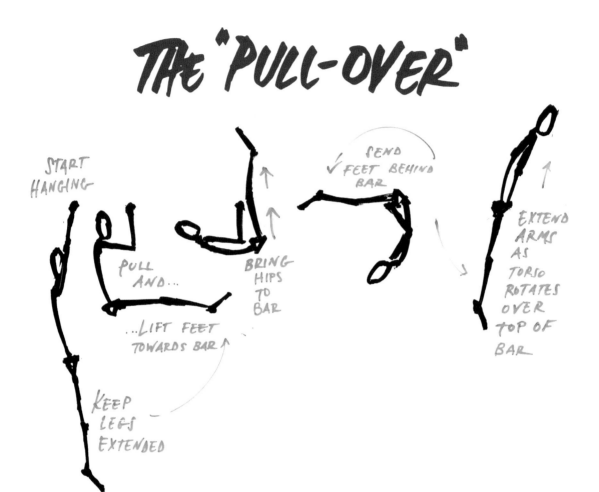

START HANGING

PULL AND...

...LIFT FEET TOWARDS BAR

KEEP LEGS EXTENDED

BRING HIPS TO BAR

SEND FEET BEHIND BAR

EXTEND ARMS AS TORSO ROTATES OVER TOP OF BAR

Points of performance

- The athlete starts with the arms extended and the hands placed on the bar just outside the shoulders.

- The legs stay extended.

- The athlete pulls with the arms and lifts the feet toward the bar.

- The athlete brings the hips to the bar and then sends the feet behind the bar.

- The arms extend as the torso rotates over the top of the bar.

PULL-UP

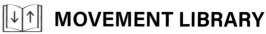

THE BUTTERFLY PULL-UP

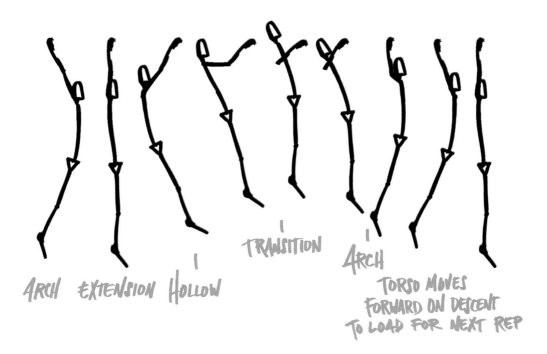

ARCH   EXTENSION   HOLLOW   TRANSITION   ARCH

TORSO MOVES FORWARD ON DESCENT TO LOAD FOR NEXT REP

Points of performance

- The hands should grip the bar just outside shoulder width in a full grip.

- The athlete starts in a hanging position with the arms extended.

- They initiate a swing with the shoulders.

- They alternate between arched and hollow positions.

- From the arched position, the athlete drives the legs toward the bar.

- At the same time, they push down on the bar with straight arms and then pull with the arms to bring the chin higher than the bar.

- The athlete allows the torso to move forward during the descent.

- The legs move back, which places the body into the arched position for the next rep.

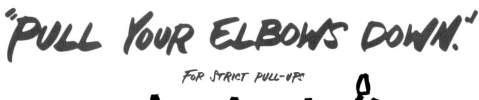

FOR STRICT PULL-UPS

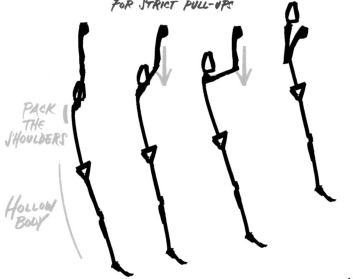

PACK THE SHOULDERS

HOLLOW BODY

Mehdi (@stronglifts)

When?

Use this cue for coaching strict pull-ups.

What does this mean?

The athlete should initiate the pull-up by retracting their shoulders and then driving their elbows down to pull themselves up.

Why?

Just as the cue "push the earth away" (pages 64 and 92) can help for deadlifts and push-ups, changing the perspective of the pull-up movement sequence by reframing it as "pulling the elbows down" can help things click for an athlete.

PUSH-UP

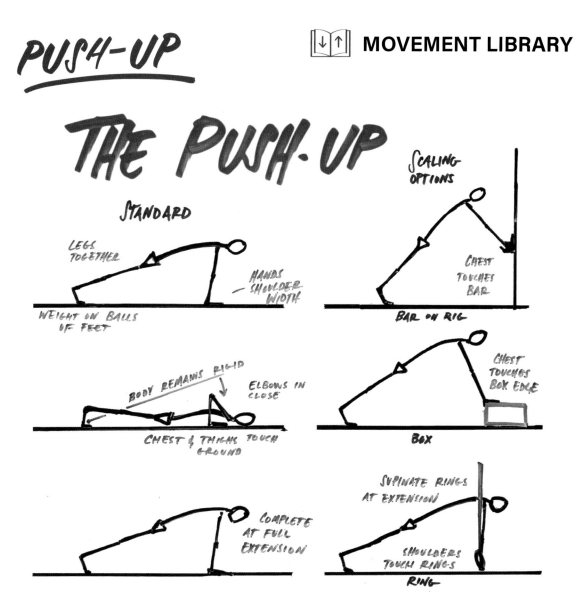

THE PUSH-UP

SCALING OPTIONS

STANDARD

LEGS TOGETHER

HANDS SHOULDER WIDTH

WEIGHT ON BALLS OF FEET

CHEST TOUCHES BAR

BAR ON RIG

BODY REMAINS RIGID

ELBOWS IN CLOSE

CHEST & THIGHS TOUCH GROUND

CHEST TOUCHES BOX EDGE

BOX

COMPLETE AT FULL EXTENSION

SUPINATE RINGS AT EXTENSION

SHOULDERS TOUCH RINGS

RING

Points of performance

- The hands should be approximately shoulder-width apart.
- The legs are together with only the balls of the feet on the ground.
- The athlete starts with the arms extended.
- The body stays rigid.
- The athlete lowers the chest and thighs to the ground.
- The elbows stay close to the body.
- The movement is complete at full arm extension.

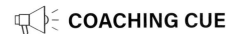

"ARROW NOT A 'T'"

ARM POSITION FOR PUSH-UPS

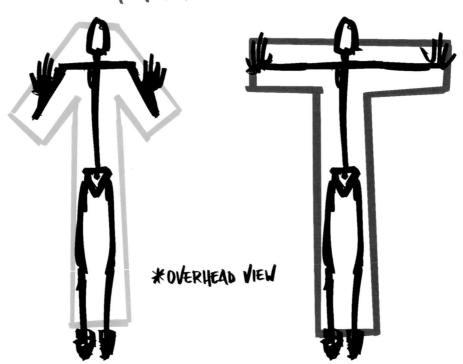

*OVERHEAD VIEW

What does this mean?

During the push-up, the aerial view of the athlete's body should imitate the shape of an arrow rather than a T.

Why?

This position is easier on the shoulder joints and allows more engagement of the back muscles.

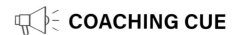
"ELBOW PITS FORWARD"

TOP OF PUSH-UP / PLANK

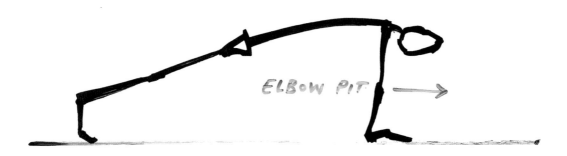

ELBOW PIT

What does this mean?

As the athlete pushes the earth away (page 64), their hands are spread wide with index fingers pointed forward. Externally rotating the hands into the ground creates torque through the arms.

Why?

This torque creates an organized position where the athlete engages the powerful lats, increasing their movement efficiency.

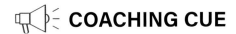
COACHING CUE

"PUSH THE EARTH AWAY"

FOR PUSH-UPS

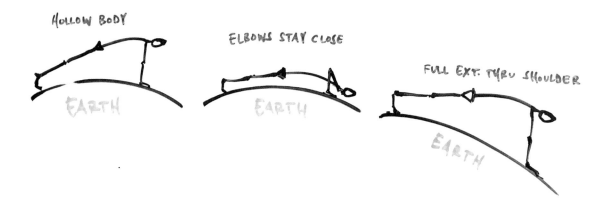

What does this mean?

Pushing the earth away is an excellent cue to emphasize how far the athlete should press through extension to the fullest range of motion of the arms and shoulders.

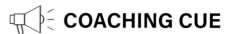

"TUCK THE BUTT"

FOR PLANKS AND PUSH-UPS

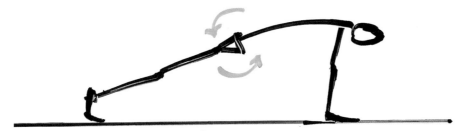

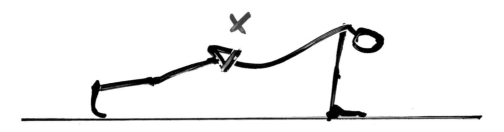

When?

Use this cue to describe creating a hollow position during planks and push-ups.

What does this mean?

When creating a hollow body position, the pelvis should have a posterior tilt. Another way to imagine this is "tucking the butt" underneath the torso.

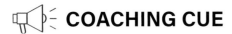
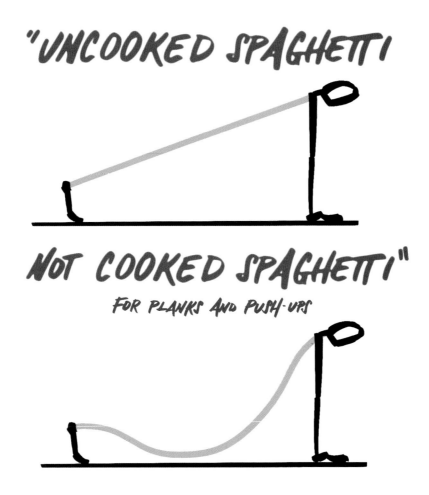

"UNCOOKED SPAGHETTI

NOT COOKED SPAGHETTI"

FOR PLANKS AND PUSH-UPS

What does this mean?

A common error during the plank and push-up is allowing the core to relax, leading to what looks like cooked spaghetti. Encourage your athlete to mimic the shape of uncooked spaghetti to keep the torso rigid and the core activated.

RING DIP

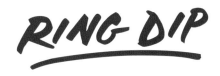

"DON'T BE A PECKER"

DURING RING DIPS

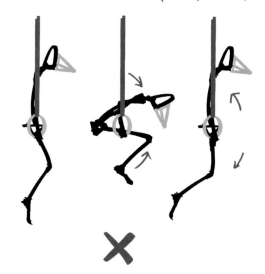

✗

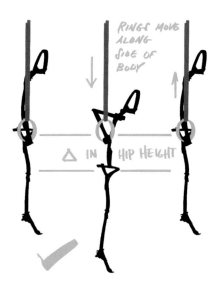

RINGS MOVE ALONG SIDE OF BODY

△ IN HIP HEIGHT

✓

h/t Travis Ewart (@travis_ewart, @invictus_gymnastics)

What does this mean?

During the ring dip, an athlete should be vertical as the rings slide up and down their torso. A common movement error is hinging at the hips and bowing forward. This resembles a bird peck. Don't be a pecker!

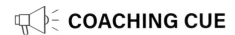

COACHING CUE

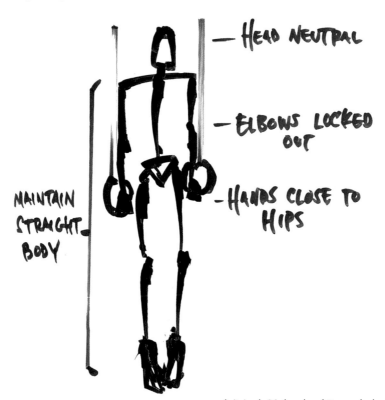

"STAND AT ATTENTION"

—DURING RING SUPPORT POSITION—

— HEAD NEUTRAL

— ELBOWS LOCKED OUT

MAINTAIN STRAIGHT BODY

— HANDS CLOSE TO HIPS

h/t Josh Melendez (@coach_josh_melendez87)

When?

Use this cue to help an athlete who's working on stabilization at the top of the ring support position.

What does this mean?

When a Marine stands at attention, they snap to a rigid torso position, with arms and hands pressed against the body.

SIT-UP

"OVERHEAD PASS"

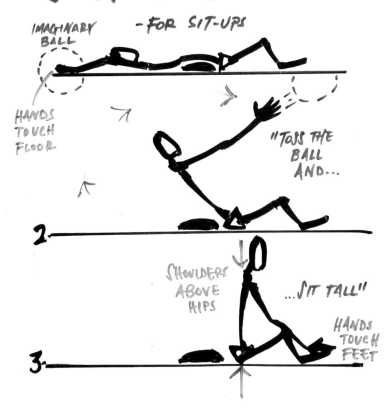

- FOR SIT-UPS

IMAGINARY BALL

HANDS TOUCH FLOOR

"TOSS THE BALL AND..."

2.

SHOULDERS ABOVE HIPS

...SIT TALL"

HANDS TOUCH FEET

3.

When?

Use this cue while demonstrating the sit-up (if appropriate for the standards for the movement in the workout).

What does this mean?

The same movement pattern used for a standing overhead pass during a sport to facilitate core-to-extremity movement can be used during this exercise.

Why?

This cue may help the athlete to understand how to use their arms during sit-ups.

T2B AND K2E

"CLOSE THE WINDOW"

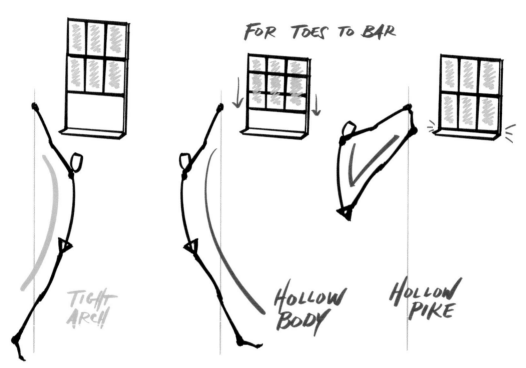

FOR TOES TO BAR

TIGHT ARCH

HOLLOW BODY

HOLLOW PIKE

When?

This cue is for doing kipping toes to bar.

What does this mean?

Have the athlete imagine they are "closing a window" (hands on a window rail, pulling down with straight arms) as they move through the hollow position in the kip.

Why?

By doing so, they will incorporate more lat activation and increase movement efficiency.

Need more help?

A great resource for this movement is the "Building Lats to Fly" program from @thebarbellphysio and @pamelagnon.

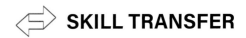
K2E ROPE CLIMB

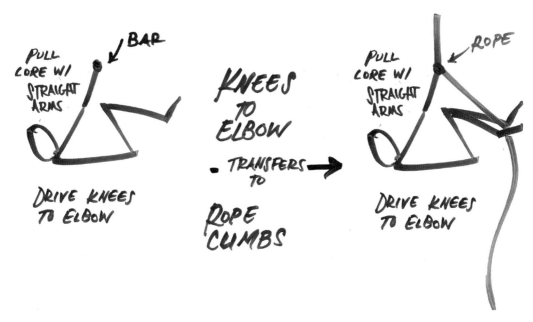

Often I see athletes struggle with rope climbs, usually from being in a more upright position on the rope and pulling with bent arms. Pulling with bent arms quickly leads to

- Arm fatigue
- Smaller "bites" up the rope
- Athlete frustration

The points of performance of the knees-to-elbow exercise are a great way to build efficiency in the rope climb. Benefits from transferring knees-to-elbow to rope climbs include the following:

- Keeping the arms straight places pulling power in the core.
- The athlete can take much larger bites up the rope when compared to pulling with bent arms.
- Larger bites mean less time under tension.

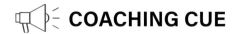
COACHING CUE

"STAY IN THE PHONE BOOTH"
DURING KIPPING TOES 2 BAR

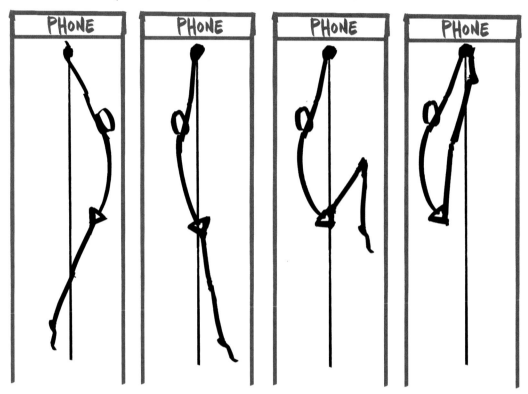

h/t Chuck Bennington
(@chuckbennington)

When?

Use this cue for kipping toes to bar.

What does this mean?

The athlete should imagine they are doing their kipping toes to bar in a phone booth, and they have to avoid hitting the walls. They should stay tight on the "toe tap" to the bar and recycle down into the next rep. Additionally, spacing should be even on each side of the bar in the hollow and arch positions.

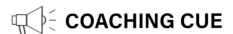
"TAP – SHOOT – RELOAD"

TO CYCLE TOES TO BAR

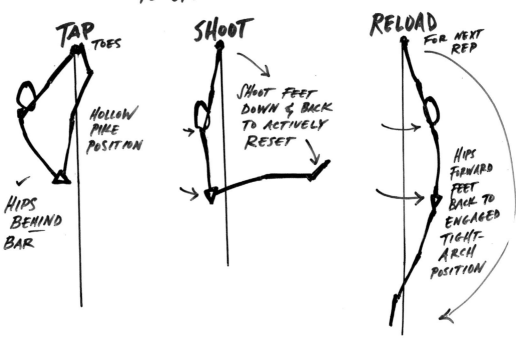

When?

Use this to cue cycling toes to bar.

What does this mean?

Once the toes tap the bar, the athlete must be in a position to actively reset ("shoot") to the arch position. This will allow them to reload for the next rep.

- **Tap:** The toes tap the bar with the hips *behind* the bar.
- **Shoot:** The legs shoot back, and the torso comes forward to *actively reset* to the arch position.
- **Reload:** The body is in the arch position with the shoulders and hips in *front* of the bar, ready for the next rep.

The same cue can be applied to the scaled movement (high-knee drive).

WALL WALKS

"DRIVE OFF YOUR KNEES"

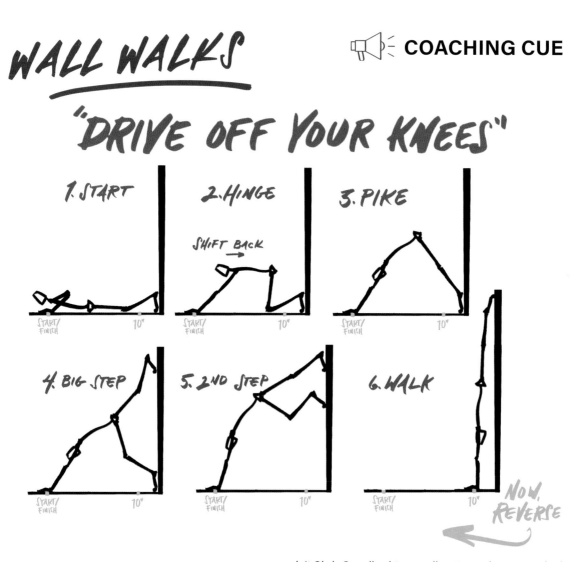

h/t Chris Spealler (@cspealler, @spealprogramming)

What does this mean?

Wall walks are a complex movement and can quickly escalate an athlete's energy expenditure. By using the following methodical approach, the athlete can move with a purpose and focus on one step at a time:

1. Press through the floor to the top of a modified push-up.

2. Stick the rear end in the air in the pike position.

3. Brace the belly and take a big step up the wall.

4. Walk the hands toward the line and the feet up the wall.

5. Reverse and bring it back down.

CHAPTER ③

DEADLIFT

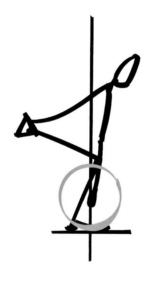

"DEADLIFT"

AKA: HEALTH LIFT, EARTH PRESS, PICKING ANYTHING OFF THE GROUND

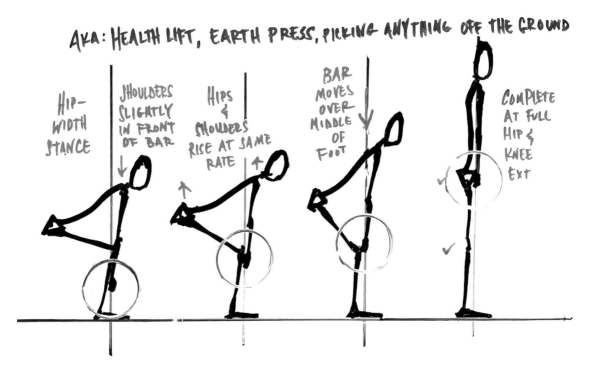

Points of performance

- The feet are in a hip-width stance.
- The hands have a full grip on the bar just outside of the hips.
- The shoulders are slightly in front of the bar.
- The lumbar curve is maintained.
- The hips and shoulders rise at same rate.
- The bar moves over the middle of the foot.
- The heels stay down.
- The movement is complete at full hip and knee extension.

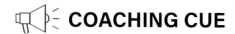

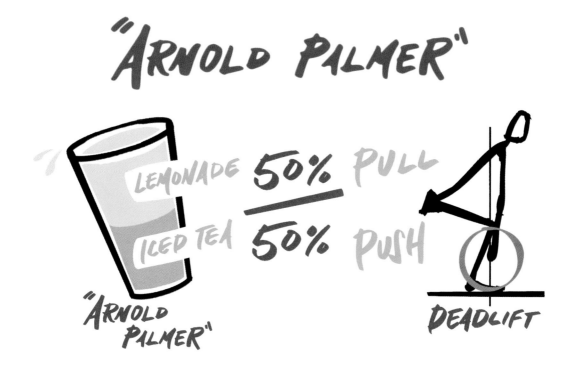

What does this mean?

An Arnold Palmer is 50 percent iced tea and 50 percent lemonade. Similarly, a deadlift is 50 percent pulling with the back and 50 percent pushing with the legs.

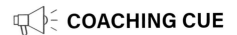

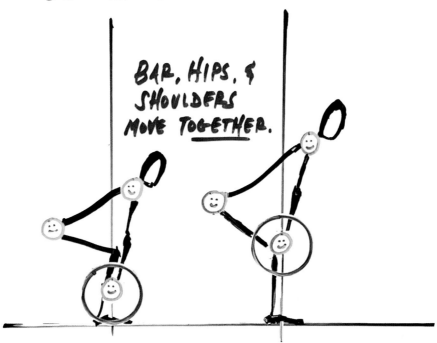

h/t the Burgener Strength (@burgenerstrength)
Level 1 Certification Course

When?

Use this cue during the first pull/ loading phase (floor to knee) of the deadlift, clean, and snatch.

What does this mean?

Throughout the loading phase of the deadlift, clean, and snatch, the bar, hips, and shoulders are the three best friends that anyone could have. They go everywhere together. They rise at the same rate until the bar is at the top of the knee.

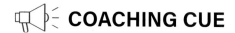
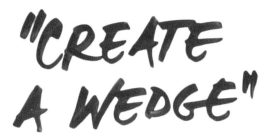

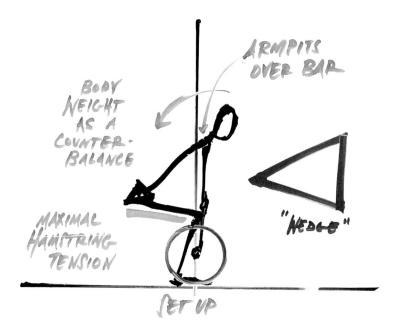

When?

Use this cue to prepare athletes to set up for the deadlift.

What does this mean?

Success with a lift begins with the setup.

When setting up for a deadlift, the athlete uses bodyweight as a counterbalance and *wedges* back. The athlete places their armpits over the bar; then they squeeze into position and slightly pull up on the bar to set tension throughout the body to be ready to initiate the deadlift.

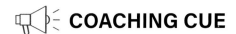 **COACHING CUE**

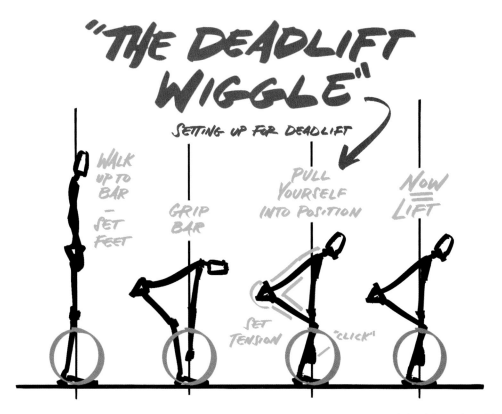

h/t Ed Coan (@eddycoan)

When?

Use this cue to prepare athletes to set up for the deadlift.

What does this mean?

As the athlete squeezes into position and sets tension through the body, they should set the grip and pull the slack out of the bar. They should find any areas where there may be slack and set tension in those areas. This will likely resemble a slight wiggle.

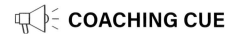

COACHING CUE

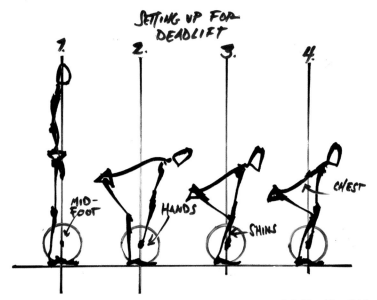

h/t Alan Thrall (@untamedstrength)

When?

Use this cue to prepare athletes to set up for the deadlift.

What does this mean?

There are five steps to a deadlift:

1. Make sure the midfoot is positioned under the barbell. *Do not move the barbell.*

2. Place the hands on the barbell. *Do not move the barbell.*

3. Bring the shins to the barbell. *Do not move the barbell.*

4. Squeeze the chest out. *Do not move the barbell.*

5. Drag the barbell up the body.

Why?

Moving the barbell prior to Step 5 will incorrectly shift the balance.

Need more help?

Watch "How to Deadlift: Starting Strength 5 Step Deadlift" by Alan Thrall at www.youtube.com/watch?v=wYREQkVtvEc.

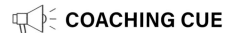
"FEEL HEAVY IN YOUR HANDS"

WHEN SETTING UP FOR DEADLIFT

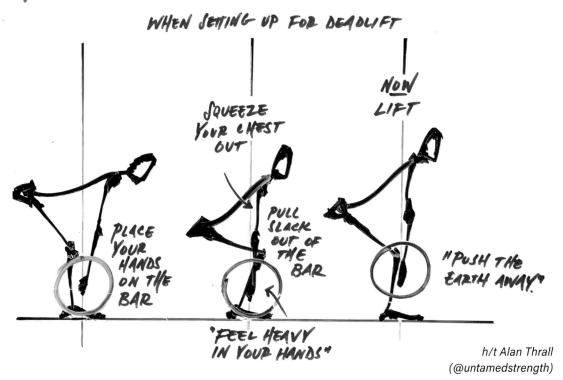

SQUEEZE YOUR CHEST OUT

NOW LIFT

PLACE YOUR HANDS ON THE BAR

PULL SLACK OUT OF THE BAR

"PUSH THE EARTH AWAY."

"FEEL HEAVY IN YOUR HANDS"

h/t Alan Thrall (@untamedstrength)

When?

Use this cue to prepare athletes to set up for the deadlift.

What does this mean?

After gripping the barbell, squeeze the chest out.

Why?

Squeezing the chest out flattens the back and straightens the arms. Consequently, the slack is pulled out of the barbell.

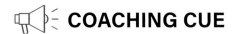
"FOCUS ON THE NEGATIVE."

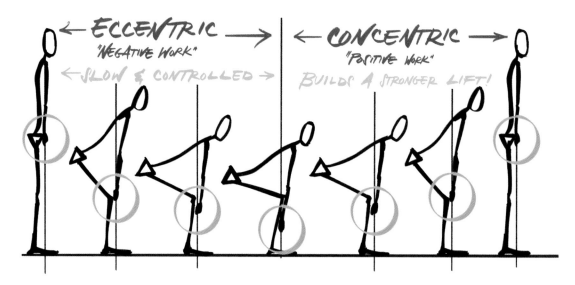

h/t Martins Licis (@martinslicis)

When?

This cue applies during the eccentric movement (the return) for the deadlift.

What does this mean?

There are two movements during a standard lift: concentric and eccentric. Concentric occurs when the muscle contracts (lifting). Eccentric, also known as the "negative," occurs when the muscle lengthens (lowering).

A common error when training the deadlift is focusing on the lifting movement and disregarding the lowering movement (the negative). Focusing on the negative not only builds strength for the concentric part of the lift but helps refine the efficiency of the bar path.

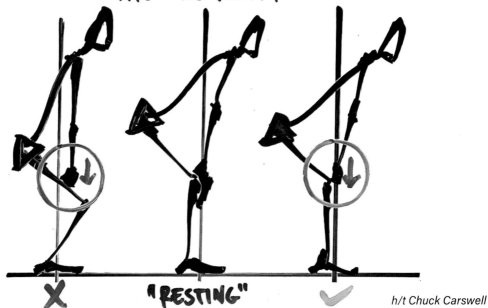

"RESTING AT THE FREE THROW LINE."

—WHEN CORRECTING IMPROPER RETURN ON THE DEADLIFT

X   "RESTING"   ✓

h/t Chuck Carswell

When?

Use this cue to help athletes correct an improper return on the deadlift.

What does this mean?

A common error when returning the bar to the bottom of the deadlift resembles a squat pattern rather than a hinge pattern.

To help an athlete understand how to move into the proper position, have them pretend they are resting at a free throw line with their hands on their knees. This will put them in a better position where their shins are more vertical and the shoulders are over the bar.

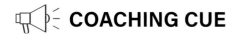
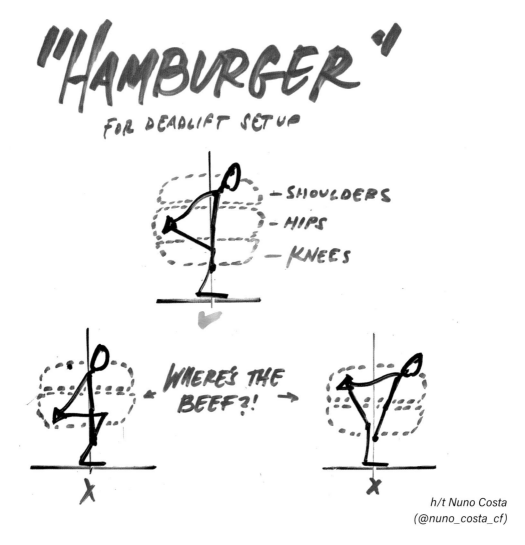

h/t Nuno Costa
(@nuno_costa_cf)

When?

Use this cue to prepare athletes to set up for the deadlift.

What does this mean?

The three layers of the body during the setup (knees, hips, and shoulders) are similar to the three layers of a burger (bottom bun, burger patty, top bun). During the setup for the deadlift, the hips should be sandwiched between the knees and shoulders.

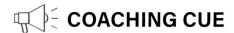
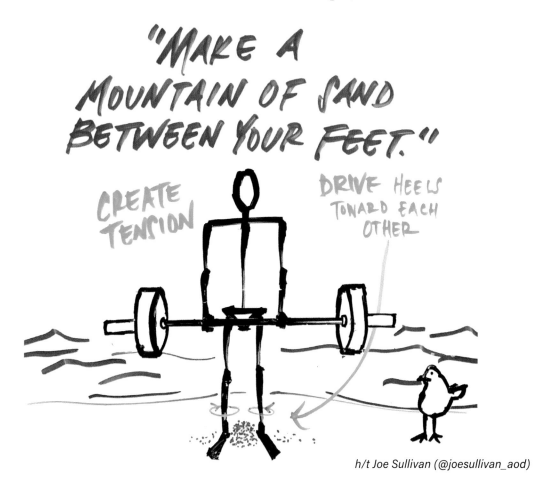

"Make a mountain of sand between your feet."

CREATE TENSION

DRIVE HEELS TOWARD EACH OTHER

h/t Joe Sullivan (@joesullivan_aod)

When?

Use this cue to coach athletes in locking out the deadlift.

What does this mean?

When driving through the lockout of the deadlift, the athlete should engage as many of their leg muscles as possible. Much of this will come from the powerful glutes, but the adductors on the insides of the legs are recruited as well. This works similarly to screwing the feet into the ground: the lifter drives their heels toward each other as if they are making a mountain of sand between their feet.

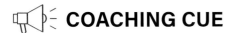

COACHING CUE

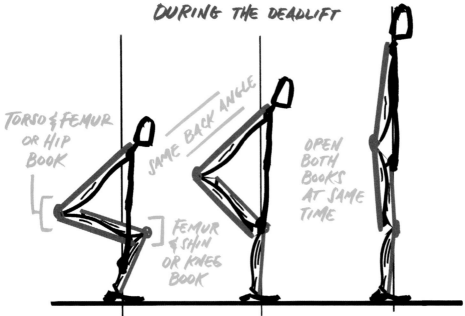

"OPEN TWO BOOKS"
DURING THE DEADLIFT

TORSO & FEMUR
OR HIP
BOOK

SAME BACK ANGLE

FEMUR
& SHIN
OR KNEE
BOOK

OPEN
BOTH
BOOKS
AT SAME
TIME

h/t Yangsu (Yu-yu) Ren (@deadlift_panda)

When?

Use this cue to coach athletes in the deadlift.

What does this mean?

Imagine the deadlift setup as two partially open books. To lift the weight efficiently, the athlete needs to fully open both books at the same time.

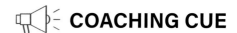
"PROUD CHEST"

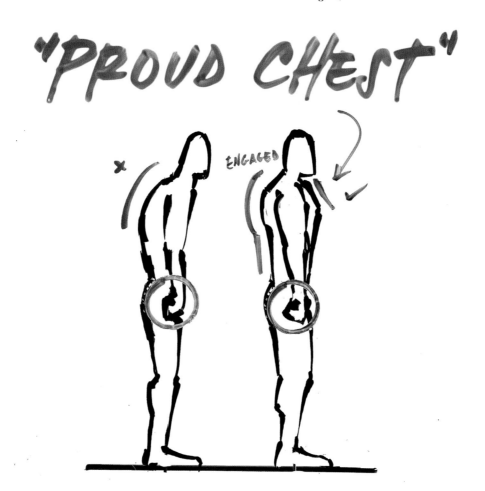

ENGAGED

When?

This cue is applicable to several situations: standing while holding a barbell at the waist, deadlift lock-out, high hang clean or snatch, and so on.

What does this mean?

Standing tall with a proud chest engages the musculature in the upper back and helps brace the core.

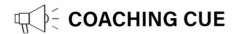

COACHING CUE

"PULL THE SLACK OUT"

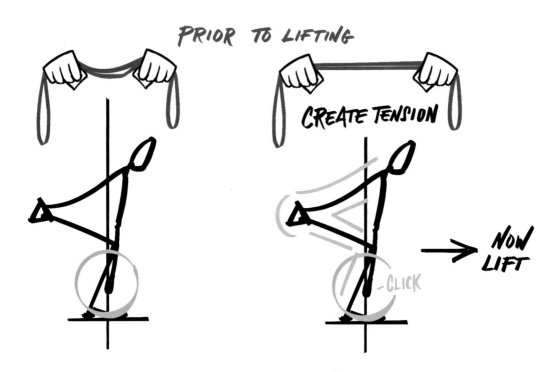

When?

This cue is appropriate before any lift in which the bar is lifted off the ground: deadlift, clean, or snatch.

What does this mean?

Once the stance, grip, and position are set, the athlete creates tension through the body by very slightly pulling up on the bar. By doing so, they take the slack out of the bar (the bend that occurs during the lift), as well as create a connection from the bar *through* the body and *into* the floor.

Why?

This simple step helps send a message from the mind to the body that says, "We are about to lift something heavy. Get ready!"

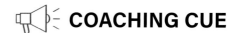

"PULL YOURSELF INTO POSITION"

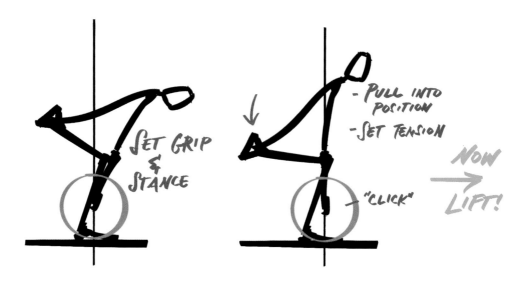

SET GRIP & STANCE

- PULL INTO POSITION
- SET TENSION

"CLICK"

NOW LIFT!

When?

Use this cue to prepare athletes to set up for the deadlift.

What does this mean?

The athlete pulls down into the starting position by taking a big breath and bracing the core. They set their grip on the bar and slightly pull up to set tension through their core and take the slack out of the bar. Once this is done, *then* they do the lift.

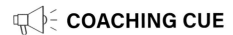
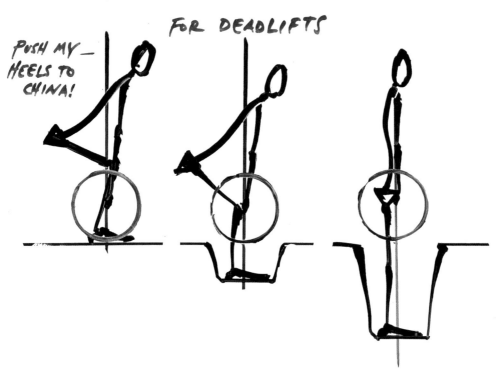

When?

Use this cue to coach athletes in the deadlift.

What does this mean?

A common mistake that novice lifters make is approaching the deadlift as if it is 100 percent pull. It is really equal parts push and pull. Cueing your athlete to push the earth away from the bar may help them engage the muscles needed to both push into the ground and pull the weight up.

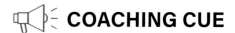

"PUT YOUR SHOULDER BLADES IN YOUR BACK POCKET."

TO CREATE TENSION FOR DEADLIFT

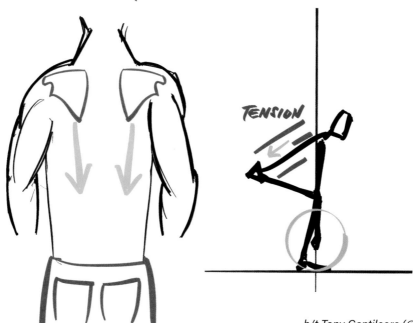

h/t Tony Gentilcore (@tonygentilcore)

When?

Use this cue to coach athletes to create tension for the deadlift.

What does this mean?

When setting up for the deadlift, the athlete should think about sliding the shoulder blades toward their back pockets. This will help properly set tension through the upper body and engage the lats.

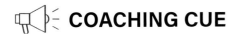
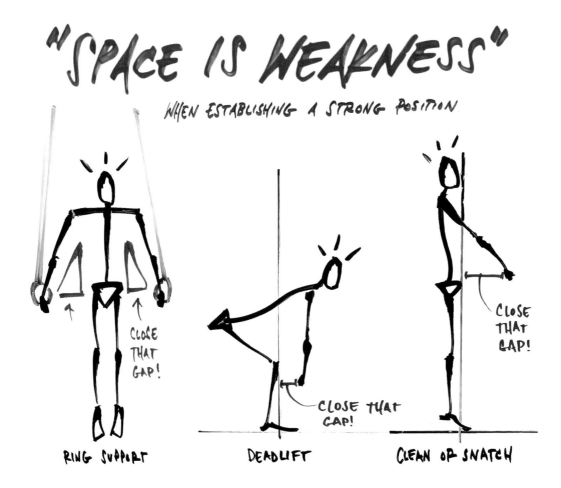

"*SPACE IS WEAKNESS*"

WHEN ESTABLISHING A STRONG POSITION

CLOSE THAT GAP!

CLOSE THAT GAP!

CLOSE THAT GAP!

RING SUPPORT

DEADLIFT

CLEAN OR SNATCH

When?

Use this cue to help athletes create a strong position for both gymnastics and weightlifting.

What does this mean?

During the ring support position, press the hands to the sides.

During the sumo deadlift, the closer the hips are to the bar, the greater the leverage.

During the clean and the snatch, keeping the bar close to the body is one of the most important factors of a successful lift.

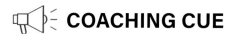
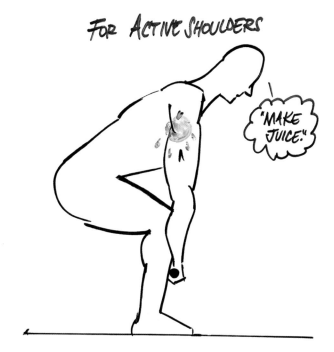

"SQUEEZE ORANGES"

FOR ACTIVE SHOULDERS

"MAKE JUICE."

via Steve Haydock (@stevehaydock)

When?

This cue is appropriate before any lift in which the bar is lifted off the ground: deadlift, clean, or snatch.

What does this mean?

Instead of saying "shoulders back," have your athlete imagine they are squeezing oranges in their armpits. You'll notice the cue to "squeeze oranges" turns the shoulders on without the risk of hyperextension through the torso.

Why?

Active shoulders are supported shoulders. Activating the lats to support the shoulders puts the athlete in a stronger position.

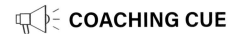
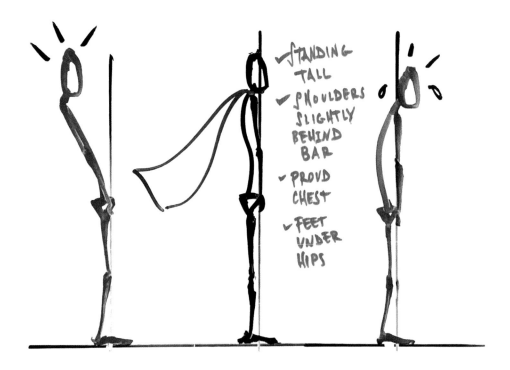

When?

Use this cue to coach the stance for the deadlift lockout or the setup for a hang clean.

What does this mean?

"Standing like a superhero" means standing tall with a proud chest and the feet under the hips.

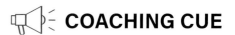

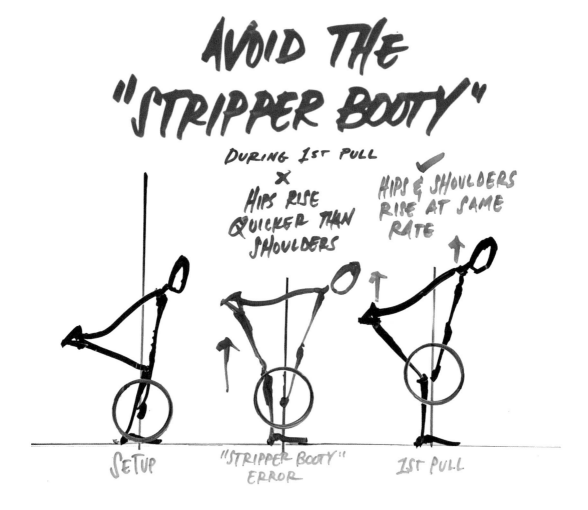

When?

Use this cue to help athletes prepare for the first pull of a deadlift, clean, or snatch.

What does this mean?

Upon initiation of the first pull, the hips often rise faster than the shoulders, placing the athlete in a weak position. However, the proper form is for the hips and shoulders to rise at the same rate, and the angle of the back should remain the same until the bar reaches the top of the knees.

Many times, the cause of this fault is the athlete rushing the first pull, which may cause the hips to shoot up first. A common fix is to slow down the first pull.

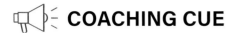
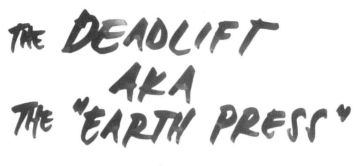

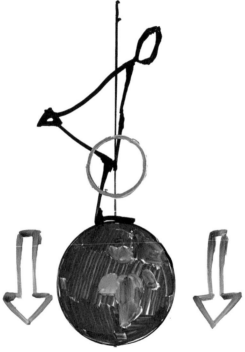

h/t Steph Earl (@stephearlstrong)

What does this mean?

Sometimes, it's all in the name. The term *deadlift* is entirely appropriate because the athlete is lifting dead weight. However, the term *earth press* is also true. The deadlift involves both pulling the weight off the ground and pressing the feet into the earth.

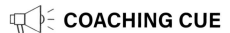

"CHEST UP, HIPS DOWN"

FOR SUMO DEADLIFT

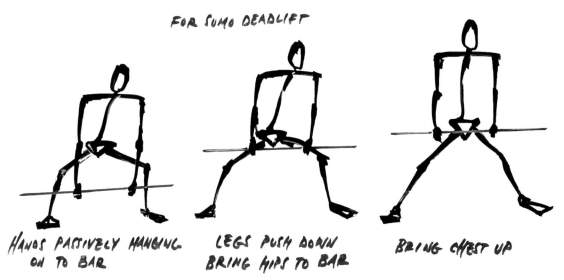

HANDS PASSIVELY HANGING ON TO BAR

LEGS PUSH DOWN BRING HIPS TO BAR

BRING CHEST UP

h/t Dr. Stefi Cohen (@steficohen)

When?

Use this cue for coaching the sumo deadlift.

What does this mean?

The athlete should focus on having their hands passively hanging onto the bar. Then they slightly pull up on the bar to set tension throughout the body and push their legs down into the floor. As their hips come closer to the bar, they bring their chest up.

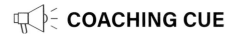

"MAKE A HOUSE"

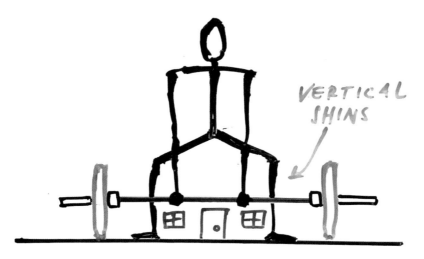

VERTICAL SHINS

h/t Joe Sullivan (@joesullivan_aod via @crossfitouest)

When?

Use this cue to prepare athletes to set up for the sumo deadlift.

What does this mean?

Make your shins vertical like the walls of a house.

CHAPTER ④

OLY LIFTING

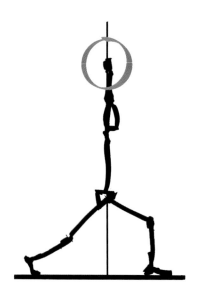

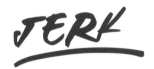

JERK

"SPLIT JERK"

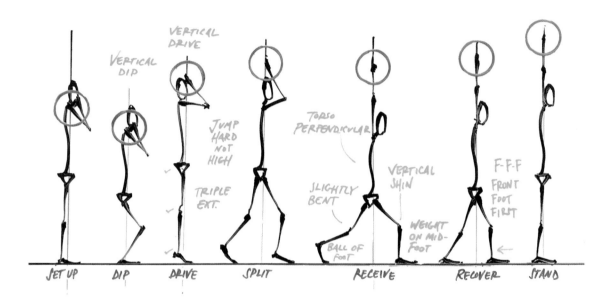

Labels: VERTICAL DRIVE · VERTICAL DIP · JUMP HARD NOT HIGH · TRIPLE EXT. · TORSO PERPENDICULAR · SLIGHTLY BENT · VERTICAL SHIN · F-F-F FRONT FOOT FIRST · BALL OF FOOT · WEIGHT ON MID-FOOT

SET UP · DIP · DRIVE · SPLIT · RECEIVE · RECOVER · STAND

Points of performance

- The feet should be in a hip-width stance.
- The hands are in a full grip on the bar just outside the width of the shoulders.
- The elbows are slightly in front of the bar.
- The torso dips straight down.
- The hips and legs extend rapidly and then press under.

- The heels are down until the hips and legs fully extend.
- The lifter receives the bar in the split position.
- The lifter brings the front foot back to center and then moves the back foot forward.
- The bar moves over the middle of the foot.
- The movement is complete when both feet are together with full arm, hip, and knee extension.

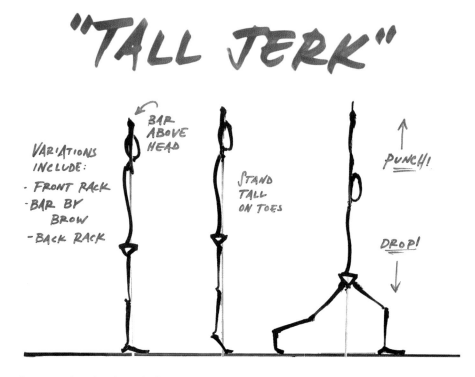

"TALL JERK"

VARIATIONS
INCLUDE:
- FRONT RACK
- BAR BY
  BROW
- BACK RACK

BAR
ABOVE
HEAD

STAND
TALL
ON TOES

PUNCH!

DROP!

There are four basic variations:

- Half-press with flat feet
- Half-press on toes (shown in sketch)
- From the shoulders on flat feet
- From the shoulders on toes

Points of performance

- The feet are in a hip-width stance with the toes turned out slightly.
- When starting from the shoulders, the bar is in the jerk rack position.
- When starting in the half-press position, the lifter presses the bar about halfway up (approximately to the top of the head) and holds.
- Without any upward drive with the legs, they lift and transition the feet into the jerk split stance, aggressively punching the arms to move down into a locked-out split receiving position.
- They lock in the overhead position at the same time the feet hit the floor.
- The lifter secures and stabilizes the bar overhead before recovering into a standing position with the bar still overhead. They move into a standing position by stepping about a third of the way back with the front foot and then bringing the back foot forward to meet it.

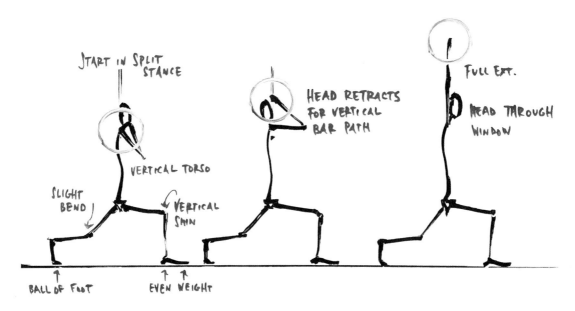

"PRESS IN SPLIT"

START IN SPLIT STANCE

HEAD RETRACTS FOR VERTICAL BAR PATH

FULL EXT.

HEAD THROUGH WINDOW

VERTICAL TORSO

SLIGHT BEND

VERTICAL SHIN

BALL OF FOOT

EVEN WEIGHT

Points of performance

- The athlete is in the split-jerk receive position with the bar in a front rack position.

- The torso is perpendicular to the ground.

- The lead foot is supporting weight in the middle of the foot.

- The shin of the lead leg is perpendicular to the ground.

- The trailing leg is slightly bent.

- The trailing foot is supporting weight on the ball of the foot.

- The lifter should set the torso upright and maintain a neutral spine position.

- They back the head out of the way.

- They press the bar in a direct line overhead to complete extension.

- They control the bar during descent onto the shoulders and never allow the bar to crash down.

Progress to the next step doesn't occur until they can control the entire ROM.

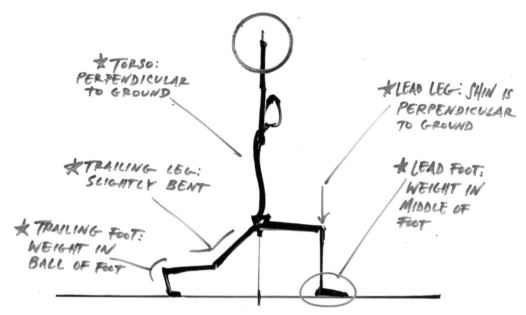

SPLIT JERK RECEIVING POSITION 5 POINTS OF PERFORMANCE

☆ TORSO: PERPENDICULAR TO GROUND

☆ LEAD LEG: SHIN IS PERPENDICULAR TO GROUND

☆ TRAILING LEG: SLIGHTLY BENT

☆ LEAD FOOT: WEIGHT IN MIDDLE OF FOOT

☆ TRAILING FOOT: WEIGHT IN BALL OF FOOT

Points of performance

1. The middle of the lead foot is supporting weight.
2. The shin of the lead leg is perpendicular to the ground.
3. The torso is perpendicular to the ground.
4. The trailing leg is slightly bent.
5. The ball of the trailing foot is supporting weight.

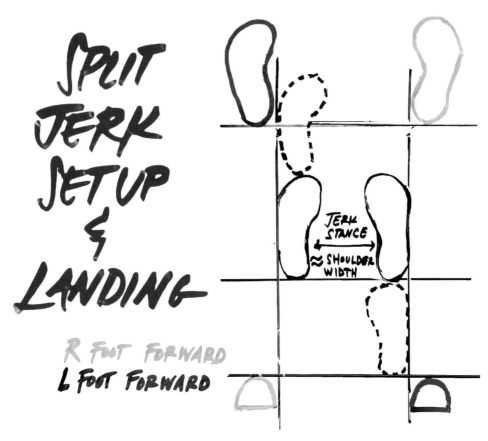

SPLIT JERK SETUP & LANDING

R FOOT FORWARD
L FOOT FORWARD

JERK STANCE
≈ SHOULDER WIDTH

adapted from the post "Split Jerk Foot Position Setup"
on the @atginsta website featuring Jami Tikkanen
(@jamitikkanen) and Mike Burgener (@mikeburgener)

When?

Prior to drilling the split jerk foot position, take a moment to draw this diagram with chalk on the platform or floor. With no bar, the athlete should practice dropping from the jerk position to the split jerk landing position. After building consistency with hitting these marks, they can progress from a PVC pipe to an unloaded bar to a lightly loaded bar, and so on.

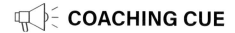

COACHING CUE

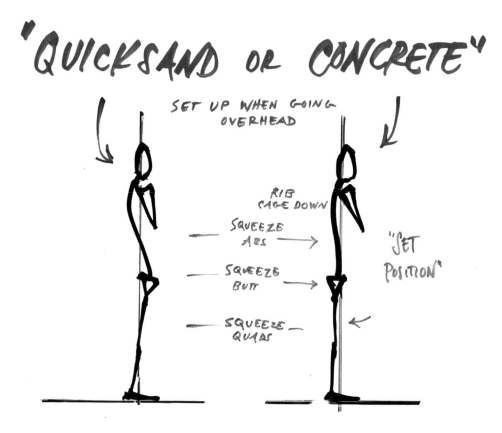

"QUICKSAND OR CONCRETE"

SET UP WHEN GOING OVERHEAD

RIB CAGE DOWN

SQUEEZE ABS →

SQUEEZE BUTT →

SQUEEZE QUADS

"SET POSITION"

When?

Use this cue for coaching athletes how to properly set up for pressing overhead.

What does this mean?

When lifting weight overhead, the athlete should have a strong foundation through the rest of the body. A loose body without much tension and with poor posture is quicksand. The athlete won't be able to transfer much power to the bar. When they squeeze the rib cage down to a neutral position and engage the glutes and quads, they create a firm foundation, like concrete. This allows them to lift and stabilize weight much better.

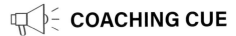
"LOAD – EXPLODE – PUNCH!"

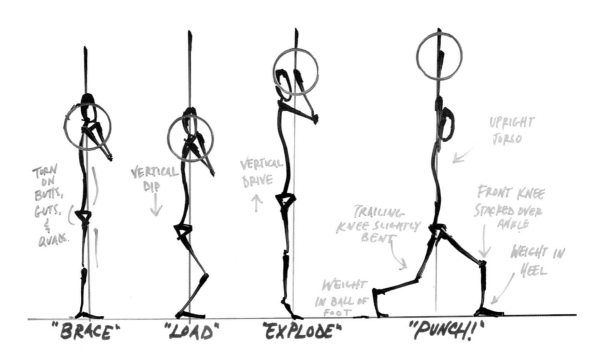

TURN ON BUTTS, GUTS, & QUADS.

VERTICAL DIP ↓

VERTICAL DRIVE ↑

TRAILING KNEE SLIGHTLY BENT

WEIGHT IN BALL OF FOOT

UPRIGHT TORSO

FRONT KNEE STACKED OVER ANKLE

WEIGHT IN HEEL

"BRACE"   "LOAD"   "EXPLODE"   "PUNCH!"

When?

This cue applies to both the push jerk and the split jerk.

Points of performance

This three-word command is a simple way to describe the movement sequence of the push or split jerk.

- **Load:** Vertical dip to the power position.
- **Explode:** Aggressive vertical extension through the hips, knees, and ankle.
- **Punch:** Punch the body under the bar, locking out the *moment* the feet connect with the ground.

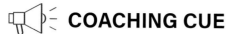
COACHING CUE

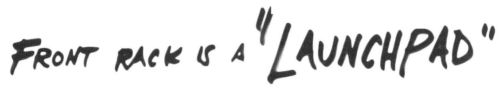
FRONT RACK IS A "LAUNCHPAD"

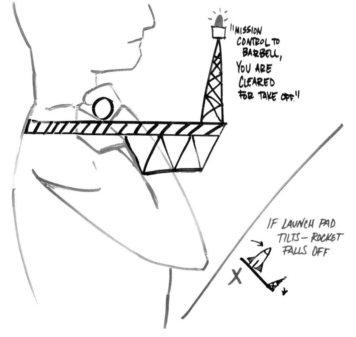

"MISSION CONTROL TO BARBELL, YOU ARE CLEARED FOR TAKE OFF."

IF LAUNCH PAD TILTS — ROCKET FALLS OFF

When?

Use this cue to coach the push jerk, push press, or thruster.

What does this mean?

The athlete should imagine the front rack is a launch pad for the barbell (or rocket):

- **Contact:** The barbell (rocket) must be in contact with the front rack (launch pad). It can't be floating out in space.

- **Vertical dip and drive:** The front rack (launch pad) must be level throughout the drive phase. If the athlete doesn't keep it level, the direction of the barbell (rocket) changes.

Why?

In the push jerk, push press, and thruster, the power generated from the hip transfers through the torso and into the bar. The front rack is the point of contact for the most efficient transfer of power, making it the launch pad for the barbell.

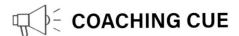

THE FRONT RACK "TRIANGLES OF SUPPORT"

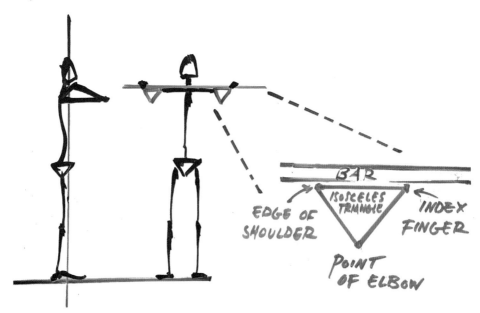

h/t Chad Vaughn (@olychad)

When?

Use this cue for athletes setting up with the barbell in the front rack position.

What does this mean?

When an athlete holds the bar in the front rack position, they want to have external rotation through the arms. The amount of external rotation needed is dependent on the elbow position in relation to the hand. Looking from the front, the elbow should be between the shoulder and the hand, creating a triangle.

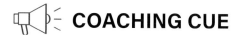

COACHING CUE

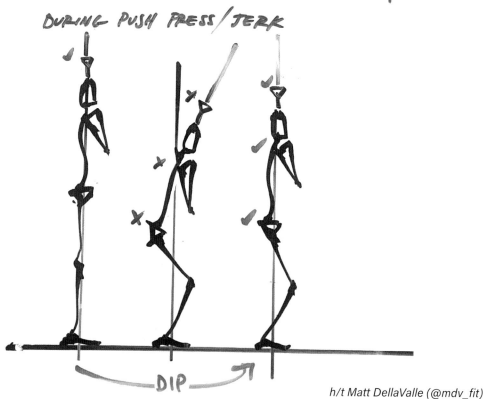

"*FLASHLIGHT ON TOP OF HEAD*"

DURING PUSH PRESS / JERK

DIP

h/t Matt DellaValle (@mdv_fit)

When?

This cue applies to the vertical dip and drive, such as in the push press or push jerk.

What does this mean?

Athletes commonly make the mistake of bowing forward during the dip. With proper form, the torso should move straight down and straight up in the sagittal plane during the dip and drive phases. In an effort to help an athlete who bows, cue the athlete to imagine they have a flashlight pointing up from the top of their head. During the dip phase, they need to keep the light shining on the ceiling.

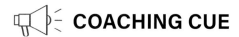
"ELEVATOR SHAFT"

FOR VERTICAL DIP & DRIVE

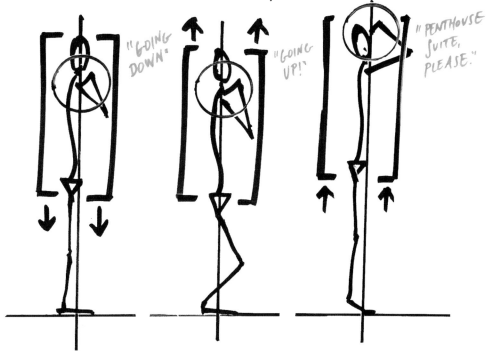

When?

Use this cue during the dip and drive of the push press or jerk.

What does this mean?

When standing in the drive position, imagine the torso moving directly up and down as if in an elevator shaft.

When?

This maintains the balance of the system over the foot and ensures the bar trajectory is up and slightly back.

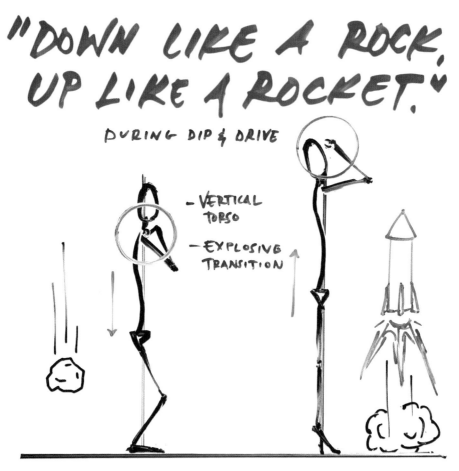

"DOWN LIKE A ROCK, UP LIKE A ROCKET."

DURING DIP & DRIVE

— VERTICAL TORSO

— EXPLOSIVE TRANSITION

h/t Wil Fleming (@wilfleming)

When?

This cue applies to the dip and drive of the push press or jerk.

What does this mean?

This cue may help the athlete understand two important concepts of the dip and drive:

- **Direction:** Like a falling rock or an exploding rocket, the direction of the dip and drive should be straight down and straight up—no leaning forward or back.

- **Speed:** A rock falls fast. A rocket travels up even faster. The transition between the dip and the drive must be explosive.

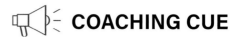

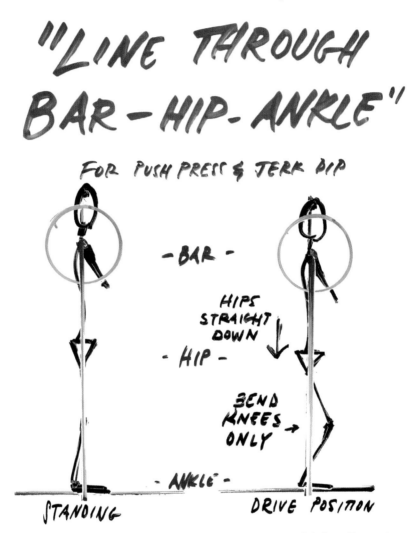

"LINE THROUGH BAR - HIP - ANKLE"

FOR PUSH PRESS & JERK DIP

- BAR -

HIPS STRAIGHT DOWN

- HIP -

BEND KNEES ONLY →

- ANKLE -

STANDING

DRIVE POSITION

h/t Greg Everett (@catalystathletics)

When?

This cue applies during the push press or jerk dip.

What does this mean?

During the drive position of the jerk or push press, there should be a vertical line running through the bar, hip, and ankle. Keeping these three points stacked helps transfer power efficiently, maintains a balance of the system over the foot, and ensures the bar trajectory is up and slightly back.

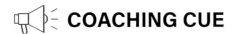
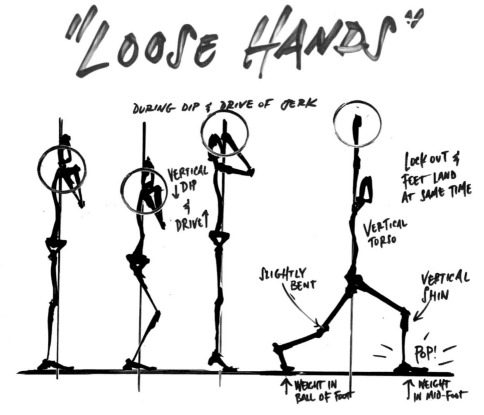

h/t Chris Spealler (@cspealler)

When?

Use this cue to prepare athletes for the dip and drive phase of the split jerk.

What does this mean?

Keeping loose hands during the dip and drive phase of the jerk may help the athlete to avoid pinning the bar to their shoulders when gripping the bar too tight.

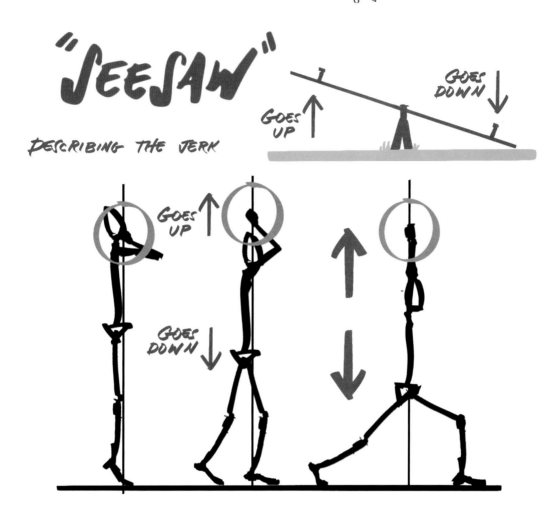

"SEESAW"

DESCRIBING THE JERK

When?

This describes the movement sequence of the jerk.

What does this mean?

One side of a seesaw rises as the other drops, and the same movement pattern happens between the bar and the body during the jerk. As the bar is launched upward off the front rack, the arms continue to push up as the body drops into the receiving position (split jerk, power jerk, push jerk, squat jerk).

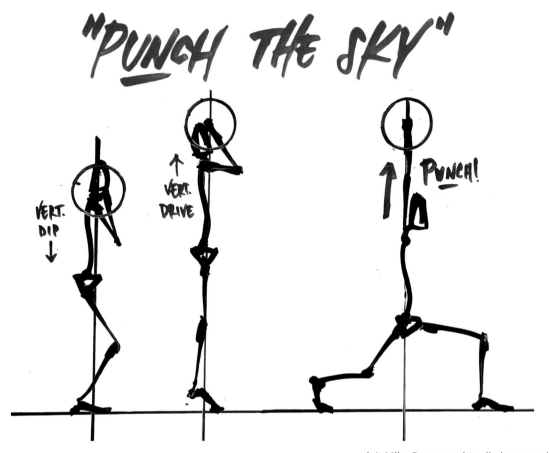

"PUNCH THE SKY"

VERT. DIP

VERT. DRIVE

PUNCH!

h/t Mike Burgener (@mikeburgener)

When?

Use this cue to remind athletes to lock out during the jerk or snatch.

What does this mean?

A common error during the jerk or snatch is to "catch" the bar on top rather than actively putting the bar where it needs to be. The jerk and snatch are anything but passive. They need to finish with an aggressive punch to the sky.

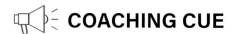
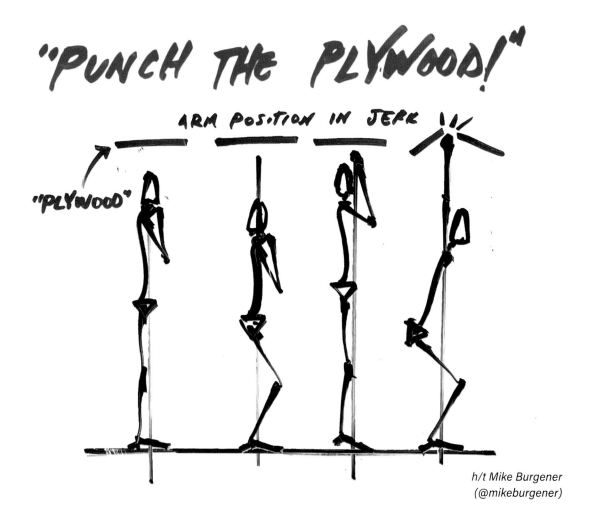

"PUNCH THE PLYWOOD!"

ARM POSITION IN JERK

"PLYWOOD"

h/t Mike Burgener
(@mikeburgener)

When?
This cue addresses the arm position for the jerk.

What does this mean?
The athlete should imagine a piece of plywood overhead as they perform the jerk. The movement of the jerk should be as if they are trying to punch a hole through that imaginary plywood, and they need to think about what position their arms would be in. The forearm position in the front rack should be the same position as if the athlete is punching straight up overhead.

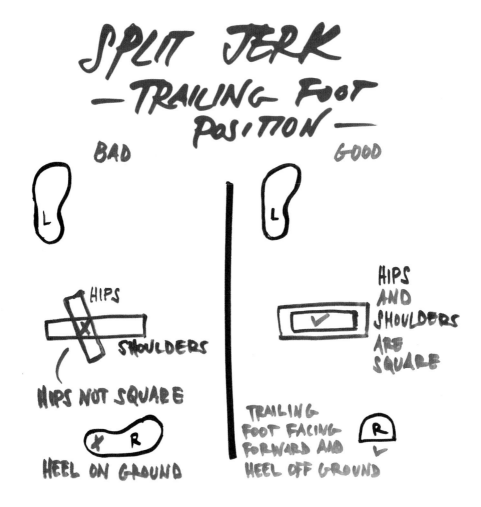

What does this mean?

A common mistake that I see with my athletes in the split jerk is in the positioning of the trailing foot. When the heel is on the ground, it pulls the hips out of alignment with the shoulders and places the athlete in a weak unstacked position. Instead, the trailing foot should be facing straight forward, and the heel should be off the ground.

A solution that may help is to suggest that the athlete "squash the bug" under the toes of that trailing foot and turn the heel out. This will allow the athlete to square the hips with their shoulders (and with the bar overhead).

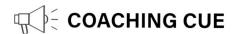
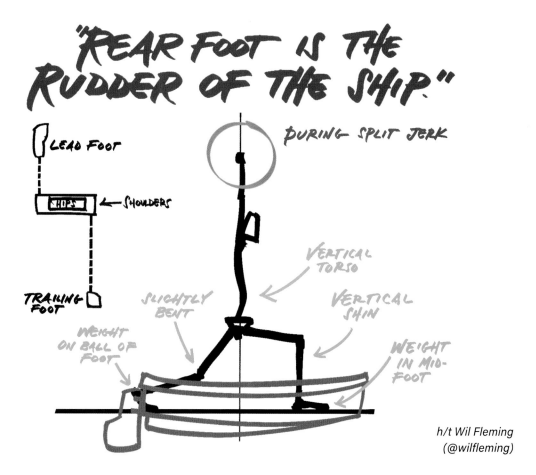

h/t Wil Fleming (@wilfleming)

When?

Use this to cue the stance for a split jerk.

What does this mean?

Much like the rudder of a ship affects the stability and direction of the ship, the rear foot plays a major role in the stability and direction of the rest of the body during the split jerk.

Note: This cue is *not* in reference to stance width.

During the split jerk, the rear foot should hit the platform a split second before the front foot. This allows the athlete to push off the back leg slightly to keep the hips under the bar as they finish moving into the split.

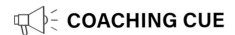 **COACHING CUE**

"RAILROAD TRACKS" NOT TIGHTROPE"

FOR SPLIT STANCE WIDTH

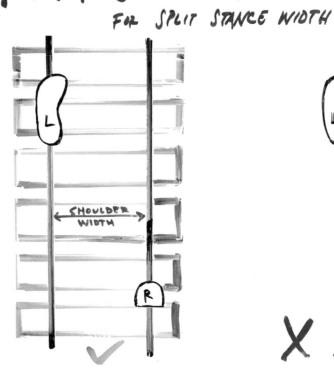

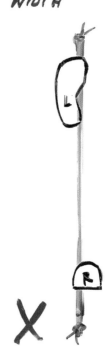

When?

Use this cue to help an athlete establish split stance width for the split jerk or lunge.

What does this mean?

When establishing a stable stance for the split jerk or lunge, the distance between the athlete's feet should be approximately shoulder width—not narrow, as if they are on a tightrope.

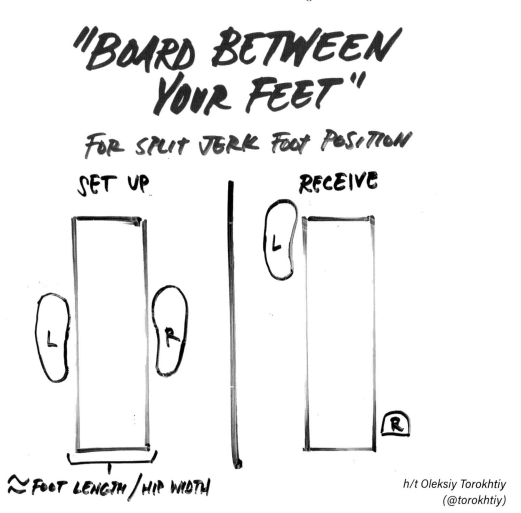

"BOARD BETWEEN YOUR FEET"

FOR SPLIT JERK FOOT POSITION

SET UP · RECEIVE

≈ FOOT LENGTH / HIP WIDTH

h/t Oleksiy Torokhtiy (@torokhtiy)

When?

This cue addresses how to establish proper foot position in the split jerk.

What does this mean?

The athlete should either imagine they're doing a split jerk with a board between their feet or practice with an actual board that's about the same width as the length of the athlete's foot. (If using an actual board for this drill, use a PVC pipe or unloaded bar.) Do 2 to 3 sets of this drill as a warm-up and another 5 to 10 reps after the workout.

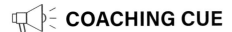

COACHING CUE

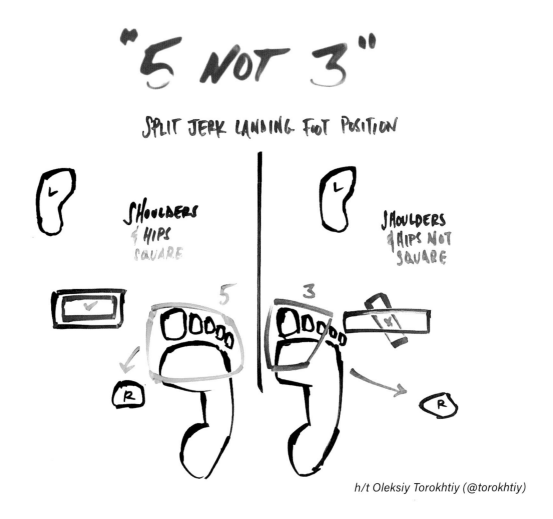

h/t Oleksiy Torokhtiy (@torokhtiy)

When?

This cue describes the split jerk landing foot position.

What does this mean?

For stability during the receive of the split jerk, the hips need to be square with the shoulders. To create this stable position, the trailing foot needs to be straight or turned slightly inward with all five toes in contact with the ground. If the foot is pointed out, with only three toes on the ground, the hips will not be square with the shoulders.

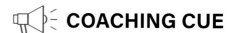
"F-F-F" FRONT FOOT FIRST

WHEN RECOVERING FROM SPLIT STANCE

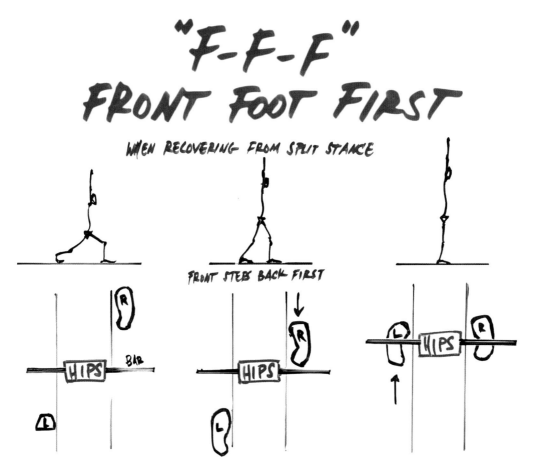

FRONT STEPS BACK FIRST

h/t Sage Burgener (@sageburgener) during the Burgener Strength Level 1 Certification

When?

Use this cue to remind athletes how to ensure a stable recovery from the split stance.

What does this mean?

The athlete should step back with the front foot first during the recovery from the split stance. They complete the recovery by stepping the trailing foot up to meet the other.

Why?

When recovering from the split stance after a jerk, stepping the front foot back first places the athlete in a stronger position to keep the weight centered over their hips and shoulders.

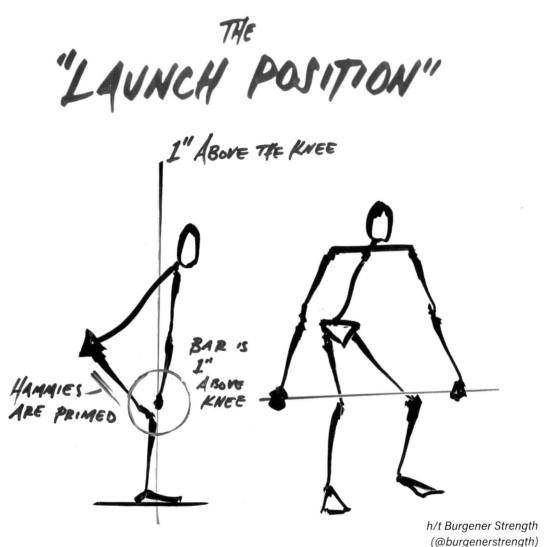

THE "LAUNCH POSITION"

1" ABOVE THE KNEE

HAMMIES ARE PRIMED

BAR IS 1" ABOVE KNEE

h/t Burgener Strength
(@burgenerstrength)

When?

The launch position is the jump sequence from 1 inch above the knee to the high hang. This position is crucial because it is the point where the hamstrings are stretched to allow for explosiveness.

SNATCH & CLEAN

THE SNATCH

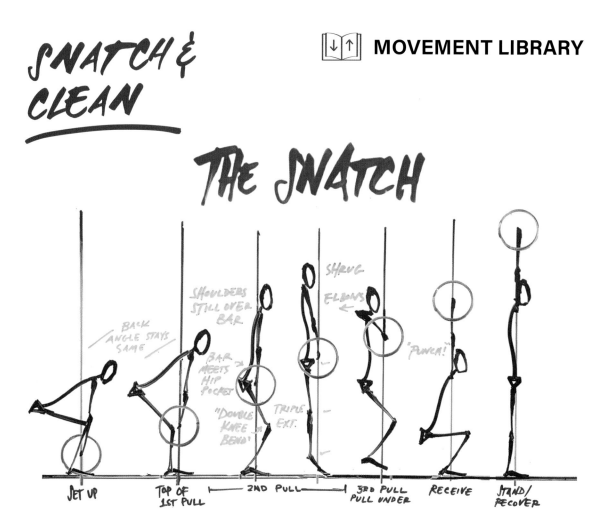

SET UP | TOP OF 1ST PULL | 2ND PULL | 3RD PULL PULL UNDER | RECEIVE | STAND/ RECOVER

Points of performance

- The athlete's feet are in a hip-width stance.

- The hands are in a hook grip on the bar at the width for an overhead squat.

- The shoulders are slightly in front of the bar.

- The lumbar curve is maintained.

- The hips and shoulders rise at the same rate, and then the hips extend rapidly.

- The shoulders shrug, and then the arms pull under.

- The athlete receives the bar in the bottom of an overhead squat.

- The movement is complete at full hip, knee, and arm extension with the bar overhead and aligned with the middle of the foot.

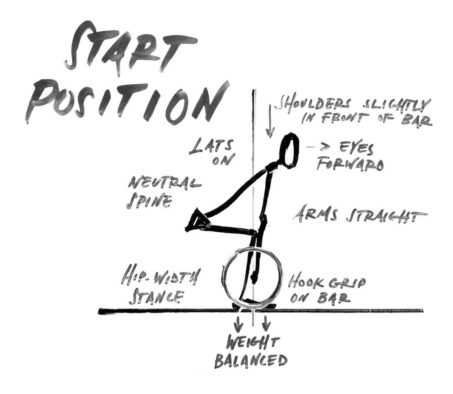

When?

These points of performance apply to both the clean and the snatch. (There may be slight differences depending on limb length.)

Points of performance

- The feet are approximately hip width apart.

- The feet are turned out 10 to 30 degrees.

- The bar is over the balls of the feet.

- The shoulders and knees are slightly in front of the bar.

- The back is set tight with a slightly exaggerated arch.

- The eyes are looking straight ahead.

Here are two differences for a clean relative to a snatch:

- The hips are higher in the jerk.

- The knees can't be pushed out as much.

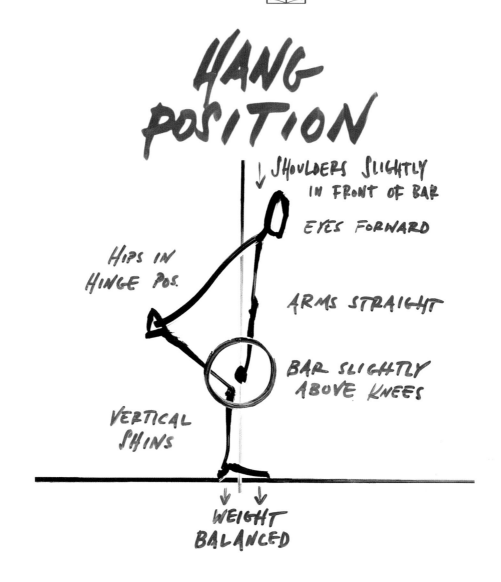

HANG POSITION

↓ SHOULDERS SLIGHTLY IN FRONT OF BAR

EYES FORWARD

HIPS IN HINGE POS.

ARMS STRAIGHT

BAR SLIGHTLY ABOVE KNEES

VERTICAL SHINS

↓ ↓ WEIGHT BALANCED

What does this mean?

The hang position is any position with the shoulders above the bar. Variations include (but aren't limited to) the following:

- Just off the floor
- Below the knee
- Above the knee
- Mid-thigh
- Power position

3-POSITION CLEAN

3 CLEANS PERFORMED
FROM 3 DIFFERENT START
POSITIONS

MOVEMENT
EXAMPLE

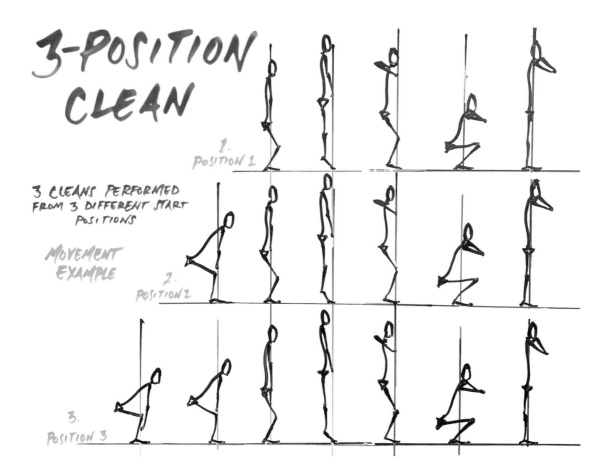

What does this mean?

The sequence of the 3-position clean may be from any of three positions desired by the coach or athlete in an effort to address a specific aspect of the lift. Most commonly, the three positions are the high hang, low hang, and clean from the floor.

THE CLEAN

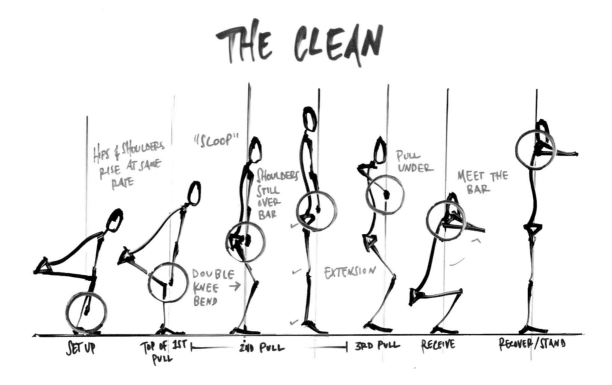

HIPS & SHOULDERS RISE AT SAME RATE

"SLOOP"

SHOULDERS STILL OVER BAR

PULL UNDER

MEET THE BAR

DOUBLE KNEE BEND →

EXTENSION

SET UP | TOP OF 1ST PULL | 2ND PULL | 3RD PULL | RECEIVE | RECOVER/STAND

Points of performance

- The athlete's feet are in a hip-width stance.
- The hands grip the bar about one thumb's distance from the hips.
- The hands are in a hook grip on the bar until the rack position.
- During the setup, the shoulders are slightly in front of the bar.
- The lumbar curve is maintained.
- The hips and shoulders rise at the same rate.
- The heels are down and the arms are straight until the hips and legs extend.
- The hips extend rapidly.
- The shoulders shrug, and then the arms pull under.
- The bar is received in a squat.
- The movement is complete at full hip and knee extension with the bar in the rack position.

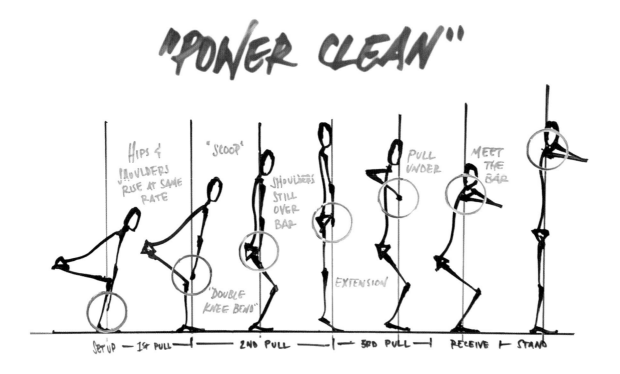

Points of performance

- The athlete's feet are in a hip-width stance.

- The hands grip the bar about one thumb's distance from the hips.

- The hands are in a hook grip on the bar until the rack position.

- During the setup, the shoulders are slightly in front of the bar.

- The lumbar curve is maintained.

- The hips and shoulders rise at the same rate.

- The heels are down and the arms are straight until the hips and legs extend.

- The hips extend rapidly.

- The shoulders shrug, and then the arms pull under.

- The bar is received in a partial squat.

- The movement is complete at full hip and knee extension with the bar in the rack position.

HANG POWER CLEAN

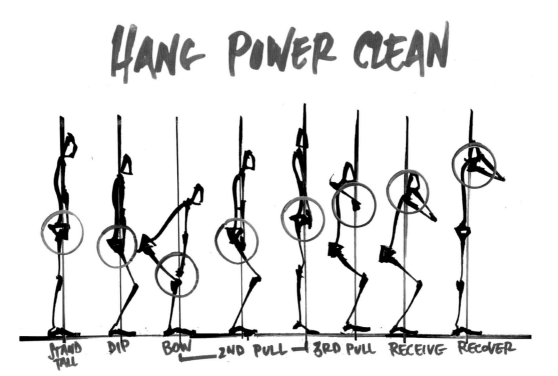

STAND TALL — DIP — BOW — 2ND PULL — 3RD PULL — RECEIVE — RECOVER

Points of performance

- The feet are in a hip-width stance.
- The grip width on the bar is a thumb's distance from the thigh.
- The hands are in a hook grip on the bar until the rack position.
- A neutral spine is maintained.
- The lifter deadlifts the bar to the hang position then hinges at the hips and maintains a neutral spine while lowering the bar to the prescribed height (see the variations).
- The hips and knees extend rapidly.
- The heels stay down until the hips and legs extend.
- The shoulders shrug, and then the arms pull under.
- The lifter receives the bar in a partial front squat.
- The movement is complete at full hip and knee extension with the bar in the front rack position.

Variations include

- **High-hang:** Upper thigh
- **Mid-hang:** Mid-thigh
- **Hang:** Top of the kneecaps
- **Knee:** Bar at the kneecaps
- **Below-knee:** Bar just below the knees

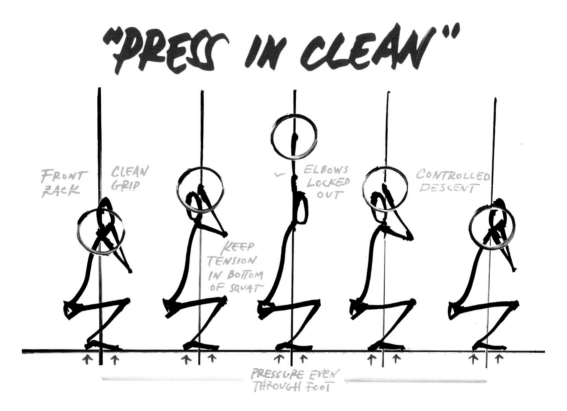

Points of performance

- The bar is in the front rack position.

- The hands grip the bar just outside the shoulders.

- The athlete is in the bottom of the squat.

- The athlete keeps tension through the core in the bottom of the squat.

- The torso is upright with a neutral spine position.

- The athlete sets their elbows under the bar.

- Press the bar overhead to complete extension.

- Control the bar during the descent onto the shoulders—never allow the bar to crash down.

Do not progress to the next step until you can control the entire ROM.

Need more help?

For more information, @catalystathletics has a phenomenal YouTube vide, "Press in Snatch (Sots Press) Mobility Progression," at www.youtube.com/watch?v=TUTFBXqEgBs.

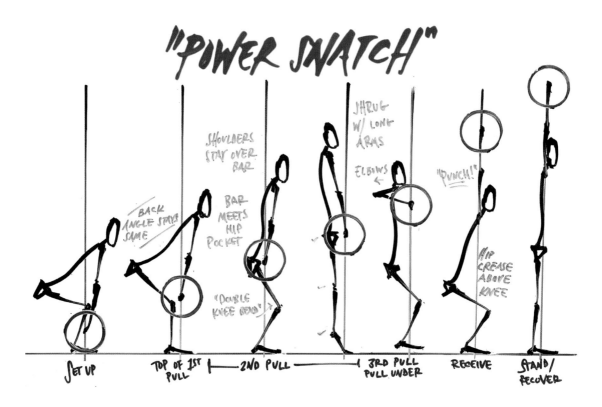

"POWER SNATCH"

SET UP — TOP OF 1ST PULL — 2ND PULL — 3RD PULL PULL UNDER — RECEIVE — STAND/RECOVER

Points of performance

- The athlete's feet are in a hip-width stance.

- The hands are in a hook grip on the bar at the width for an overhead squat.

- The shoulders are slightly in front of the bar.

- The lumbar curve is maintained.

- The hips and shoulders rise at the same rate, and then the hips extend rapidly.

- The shoulders shrug, and then the arms pull under.

- The athlete receives the bar in a partial squat.

- The movement is complete at full hip, knee, and arm extension with the bar over the middle of the foot.

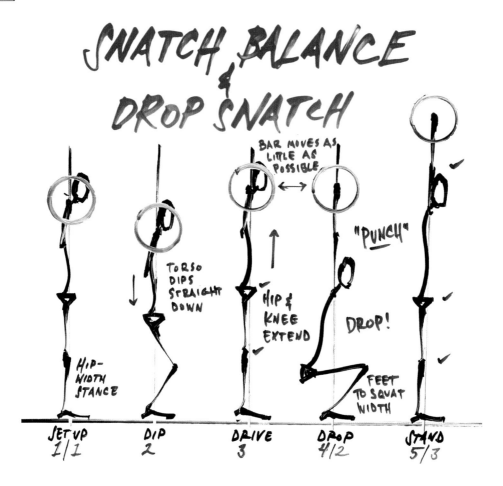

SNATCH BALANCE & DROP SNATCH

Points of performance

- The lifter's feet are in a hip-width stance.
- The bar rests on the upper back.
- The lifter grips the bar using the grip for an overhead squat.
- The torso dips straight down.
- The hips and legs extend rapidly.
- The lifter punches under so the bar moves as little as possible.

Note: There is no dip and drive for the drop snatch—only a quick drop.

- The feet move to a squat-width stance.
- The lifter receives the bar at the bottom of the overhead squat.
- The movement is complete at full hip, knee, and arm extension.

"PRESS IN SNATCH"

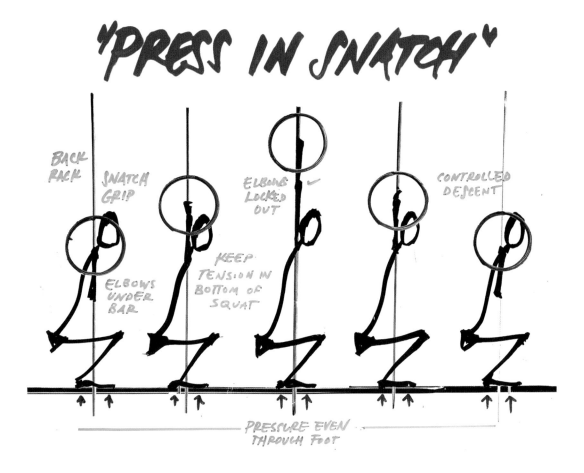

BACK RACK

SNATCH GRIP

ELBOWS UNDER BAR

ELBOWS LOCKED OUT

KEEP TENSION IN BOTTOM OF SQUAT

CONTROLLED DESCENT

PRESSURE EVEN THROUGH FOOT

Points of performance

- The bar is in the back rack position.

- The hands grip the bar at snatch grip width.

- The athlete is in the bottom of the squat.

- Tension is maintained through the core in the bottom of the squat.

- The torso is upright, and the neutral spine position is maintained.

- The elbows are set under the bar.

- The athlete presses the bar overhead to complete the extension.

- The descent of the bar is controlled down onto the back rack; it should never crash down.

- No weight is added until the athlete can control the entire range of motion.

CUES
SPEED

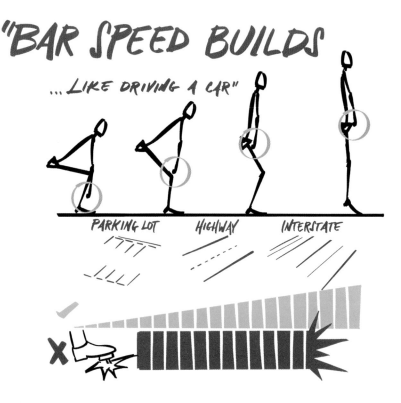

"BAR SPEED BUILDS
... *LIKE DRIVING A CAR*"

PARKING LOT   HIGHWAY   INTERSTATE

When?

Use this cue when working with athletes on bar speed for both the snatch and the clean.

What does this mean?

You wouldn't just hop in your car and slam on the gas. You start slowly and progressively get faster. The principles of driving a car also apply for pulling the bar off the ground in the Olympic lifts:

- You maneuver through the parking lot (mid-shin to above the knee).

- Then you progress onto the highway (above the knee to the hip pocket).

- Then you take the on-ramp for the interstate (hip pocket to extension).

Bar speed *builds* throughout the pull.

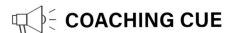

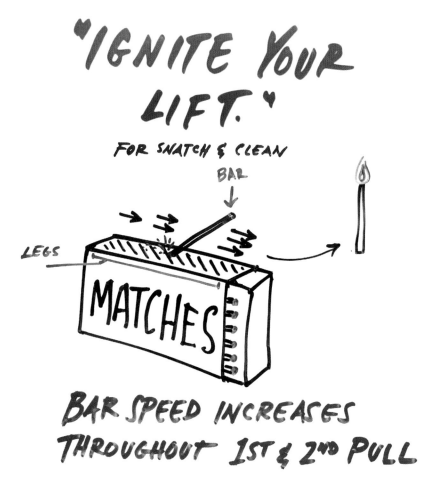

h/t CrossFit BBN (@crossfitbbn)

When?

This cue applies to the first and second pulls of the snatch and clean.

What does this mean?

As a match slides along the igniter strip, it gains speed. Similarly, bar speed should increase throughout the first and second pulls.

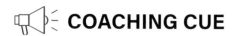 **COACHING CUE**

SET UP

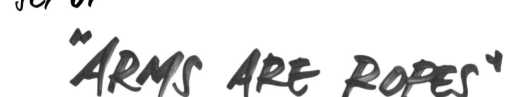

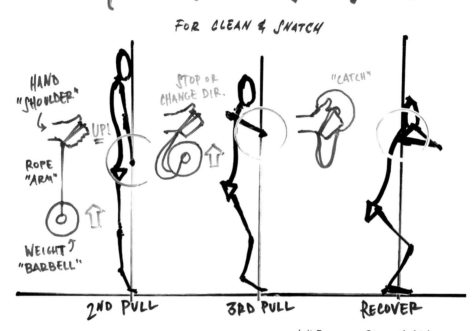

h/t Burgener Strength (@burgenerstrength)

When?

Use this cue to coach athletes during the down and finish of both the clean and the snatch.

What does this mean?

The shrug at the top of the second pull initiates the third pull and is a signal to pull the body under the barbell as fast as possible. Throughout the first and second pull of the clean and snatch, the arms are like ropes, hanging long and relaxed next to the body. Arms do not bend until after the jump and shrug.

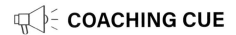
"ELBOWS OUT"

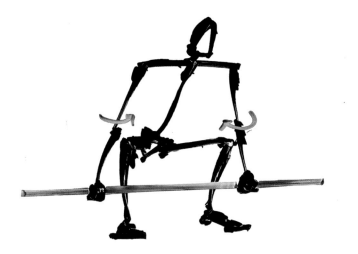

h/t Greg Everett (@catalystathletics)

When?

This cue applies to the setup for the snatch and clean.

What does this mean?

To keep the bar close to the body throughout the third pull of the snatch or clean, the elbows should drive high and back. Internally rotating the elbows during the setup will help optimize the mechanics of the third pull. Have the athlete try this:

- Stand neutral while holding a PVC pipe at the waist with either the clean or snatch grip.

- Internally rotate the arms (point the elbows out) and move them high and back, keeping the bar close to the body.

Have the athlete compare this to a neutral or external rotation of the arms. They should notice a difference.

> *"When establishing this elbow position, bear in mind that rotation of the arm is independent of the shoulder blades. Do not roll the shoulders forward attempting to create more rotation of the arm."*

—Greg Everett

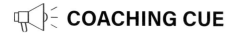 **COACHING CUE**

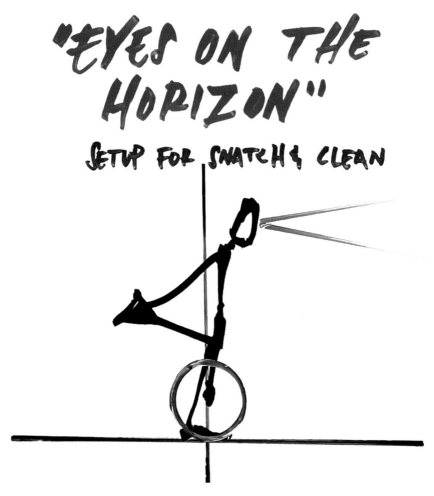

When?

This cue applies to the setup for the snatch and clean.

What does this mean?

During the set-up for the snatch and clean, the gaze should be directed toward the horizon, rather than at the floor. Looking toward the horizon helps the lifter set an optimal position by maintaining or slightly exaggerating the lumbar curve and flattening the thoracic curve. Also, keeping the eyes fixed on a single point on the horizon allows the lifter to focus on their movement, rather than being distracted as their eyes move around.

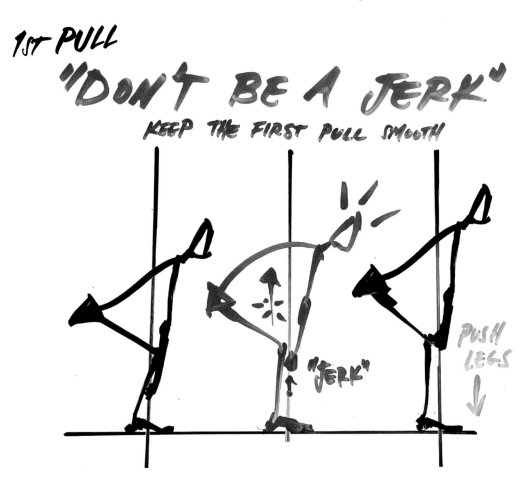

1ST PULL

"DON'T BE A JERK"

KEEP THE FIRST PULL SMOOTH

"JERK"

PUSH LEGS

When?

This cue applies to initiating the first pull of the clean or snatch.

What does this mean?

The first pull doesn't involve *jerking* the bar off the ground. The initial speed of the bar off the ground should be smooth to place the athlete in a better position to build speed throughout the first and second pulls.

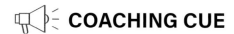 **COACHING CUE**

2ND PULL

"A BRUSH NOT A BANG"

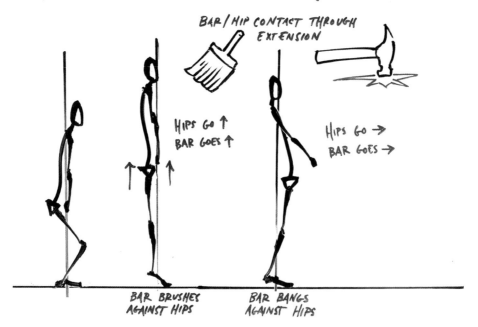

BAR/HIP CONTACT THROUGH EXTENSION

HIPS GO ↑
BAR GOES ↑

HIPS GO →
BAR GOES →

BAR BRUSHES AGAINST HIPS

BAR BANGS AGAINST HIPS

h/t Voodoo Weightlifting (@voodooweightlifting)

When?

Use this cue to describe hip contact with the bar during extension of the clean or snatch.

What does this mean?

During extension of the clean or snatch, the bar should *brush* up the hips rather than *bang* against the hips.

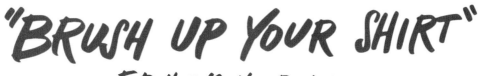

"BRUSH UP YOUR SHIRT"
FOR HITTING HIP POCKET

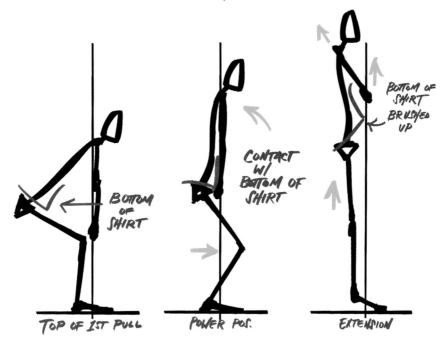

TOP OF 1ST PULL   POWER POS.   EXTENSION

BOTTOM OF SHIRT

CONTACT W/ BOTTOM OF SHIRT

BOTTOM OF SHIRT BRUSHED UP

When?

This cue reminds the athlete to hit/brush the hip pocket during the clean and snatch.

What does this mean?

During the second pull of the clean and snatch, the bar will brush up against the body (hips in the snatch, upper thigh in the clean). Prior to contact, the bar should be as close to the body as possible without dragging. This will likely brush up the bottom of the athlete's shirt.

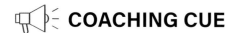

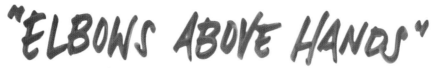

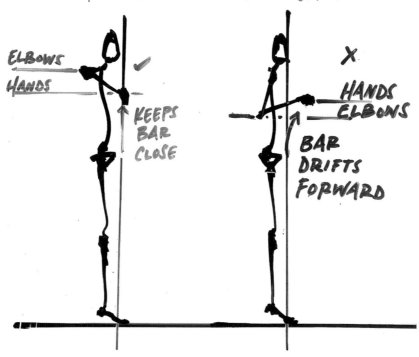

When?

This cue applies through the second pull of the clean or snatch.

What does this mean?

Throughout the second pull, the elbows should be higher than the hands. This will help keep the bar close to the body.

"FINISH THE PULL"

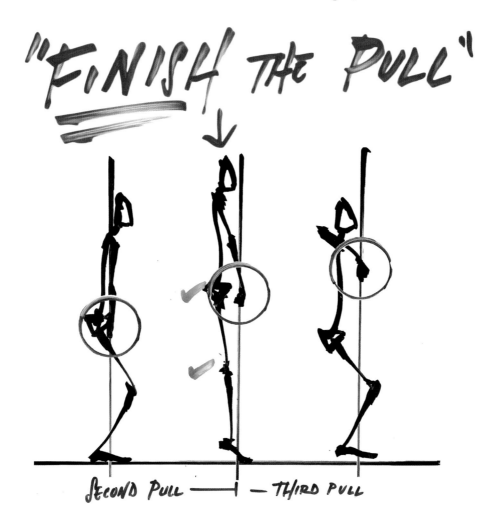

SECOND PULL ——⊢— THIRD PULL

When?

Use this cue if an athlete fails to reach full extension of their hips and knees during the second pull of the snatch or clean. Signs of this issue may include

- Jumping and landing forward when receiving the bar
- Missing the lift with the weight forward

What does this mean?

The second pull finishes with full extension of the hips and knees.

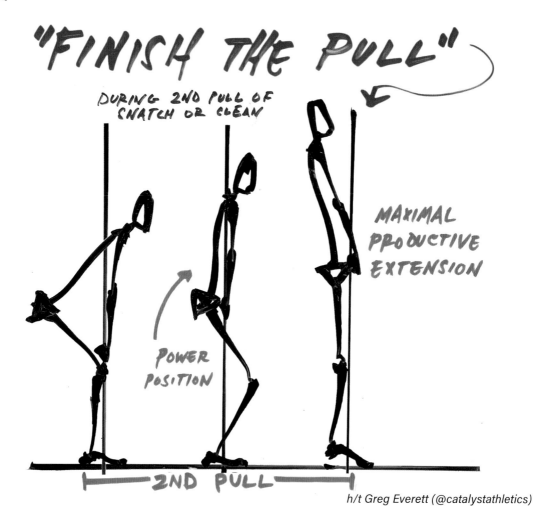

"FINISH THE PULL"

DURING 2ND PULL OF SNATCH OR CLEAN

MAXIMAL PRODUCTIVE EXTENSION

POWER POSITION

2ND PULL

h/t Greg Everett (@catalystathletics)

What does this mean?

In the final position of the second pull, the legs are vertically extended and the shoulders are behind the hips. This allows the bar to continue its vertical trajectory.

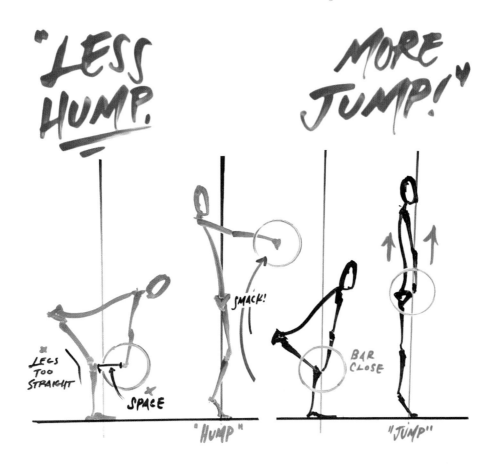

What does this mean?

A common error during the second pull of the clean and snatch is "humping," or banging the bar forward. This is normally caused by poor timing and/or too much space between the bar and body prior to contact.

The bar should brush *up* the body through the second pull. Thinking of the second pull as a jump rather than a hump may help fix the issue.

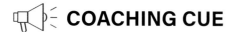
COACHING CUE

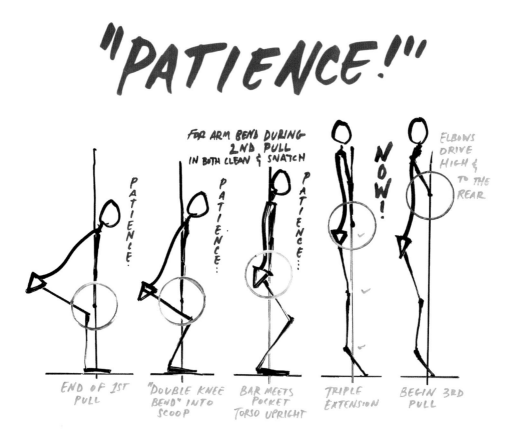

"PATIENCE!"

FOR ARM BEND DURING
2ND PULL
IN BOTH CLEAN & SNATCH

PATIENCE.

PATIENCE..

PATIENCE...

NOW!

ELBOWS
DRIVE
HIGH &
TO THE
REAR

END OF 1ST
PULL

"DOUBLE KNEE
BEND" INTO
SCOOP

BAR MEETS
POCKET
TORSO UPRIGHT

TRIPLE
EXTENSION

BEGIN 3RD
PULL

What does this mean?

A common fault in the second pull of the clean and snatch is extension of the hips prior to the bar making contact with the body. The athlete must have patience in lengthening their pull by keeping their shoulders over the bar and allowing their legs to drive into extension prior to pulling their body under.

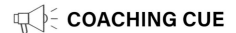

ARE YOU A PATIENT LIFTER?

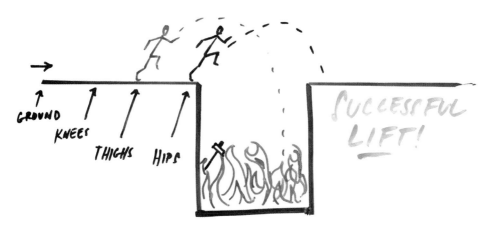

GROUND KNEES THIGHS HIPS SUCCESSFUL LIFT!

BE PATIENT. GET THE BAR TO YOUR HIPS.

h/t Christian Harris (@iamchrisharris)

When?

Use this cue to help athletes with the timing for the clean and snatch.

What does this mean?

The timing of the "jump" plays a big part in the success of the lift. Jumping too early (extending the hips prior to making contact with the bar against the hips [for snatch] or upper thigh [for clean]) will cause the athlete to miss the bar in front.

📢 COACHING CUE

"PLANE ON THE RUNWAY."

FINISHING THE PULL DURING CLEAN & SNATCH

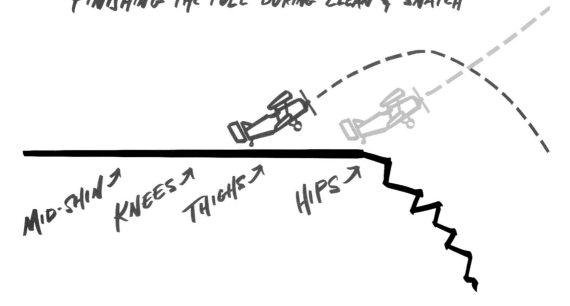

When?

Use this cue if the athlete is having a problem finishing their pull on the clean or snatch.

What does this mean?

Compare the bar path along the body to a runway. A plane needs the entire length of the runway to take off with full power. Similarly, the path of the bar should go all the way to the hips during the pull for a clean or snatch.

Why?

Not finishing the pull leaves power on the table and may send the trajectory of the bar path out in front of the athlete.

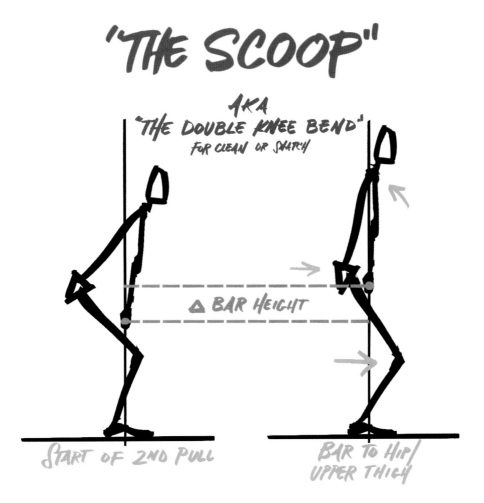

"THE SCOOP"

AKA
"THE DOUBLE KNEE BEND"
FOR CLEAN OR SNATCH

△ BAR HEIGHT

START OF 2ND PULL

BAR TO HIP/
UPPER THIGH

What does this mean?

The double knee bend naturally occurs during the second pull of the clean and snatch. The knees extend during the initial drive through the floor during the first pull. As the bar continues its upward path over the midfoot, the knees move forward. This places the lifter in the optimal position to jump up with the bar once it reaches the hip.

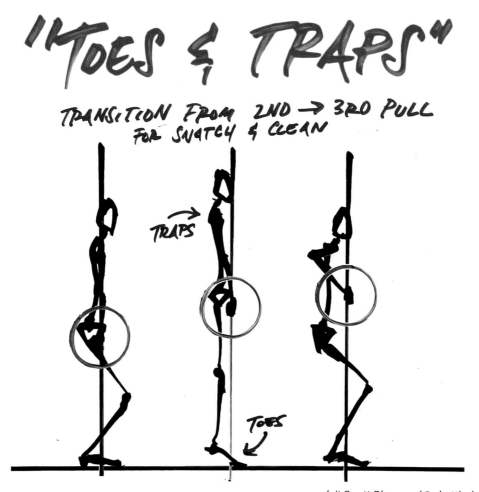

h/t Scott Pherson (@skottiedoesntno)

What does this mean?

During the clean and the snatch, "toes and traps" marks the transition from the second pull (extension through hips and knees) to the third pull (pull under the bar).

- **Toes:** When driving up into the finish of the second pull, the lifter should extend up to the top of the foot (the toes).
- **Traps:** The lifter squeezes the shoulder blades together rather than straight up.

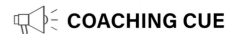
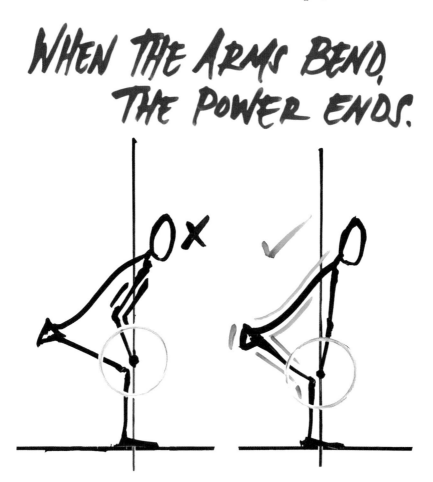

What does this mean?

If the arms bend prior to hip extension in the clean or snatch, the weight of the bar is transferred to the arms rather than the major muscle groups of the core and legs, resulting in a loss of power.

3RD PULL

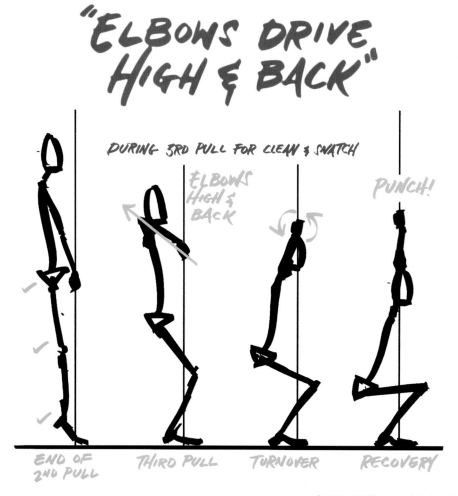

"ELBOWS DRIVE HIGH & BACK"

DURING 3RD PULL FOR CLEAN & SNATCH

ELBOWS HIGH & BACK

PUNCH!

END OF 2ND PULL   THIRD PULL   TURNOVER   RECOVERY

h/t Scott Pherson (@skottiedoesntno)

Why?

Driving the elbows high and back helps keep the barbell close to the shoulders.

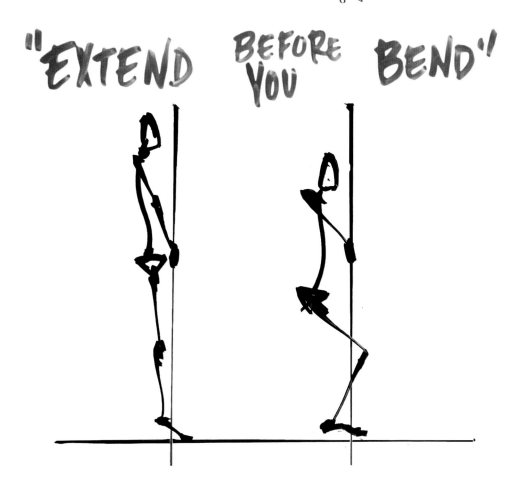

"EXTEND BEFORE YOU BEND"

What does this mean?

This phrase may help communicate the sequence of extension and flexion of the hip and knee through the second and third pulls of the snatch or clean.

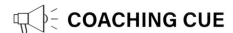
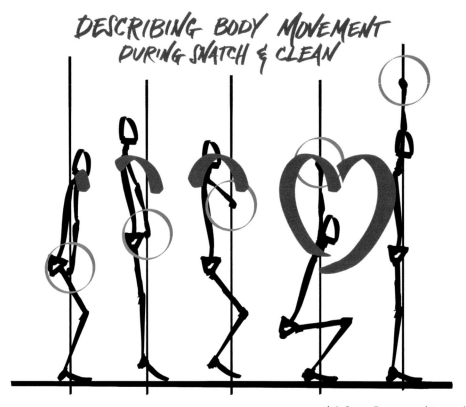

h/t Sage Burgener (@sageburgener)

What does this mean?

For the bar to travel vertically in a straight path during both the clean and the snatch, the body (specifically the shoulders) must move in a "half heart"–shaped path.

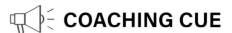

"BAR IS PIVOT POINT"
DURING TURNOVER IN CLEAN

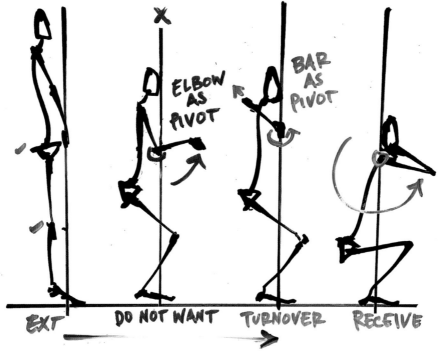

h/t Greg Everett (@catalystathletics)

When?
Use this cue to coach the turnover of the clean.

What does this mean?
When the bar is the pivot point for the clean turnover, the elbows rotate *around* the bar while the bar is kept close to the body.

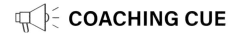

COACHING CUE

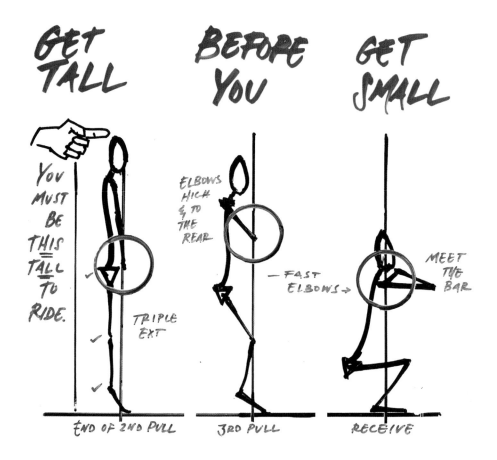

When?

Use this cue to help athletes who are having trouble reaching full extension at the end of the second pull of a clean or snatch to transition from triple extension to receiving the bar.

What does this mean?

Place your hand 2 inches above the athlete's head when they are standing tall. Cue them to touch your hand with the top of their head when they move through the clean or snatch with a PVC pipe. They'll need to reach full extension to make contact.

Why?

Not reaching full extension leaves power on the table.

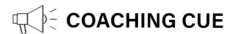
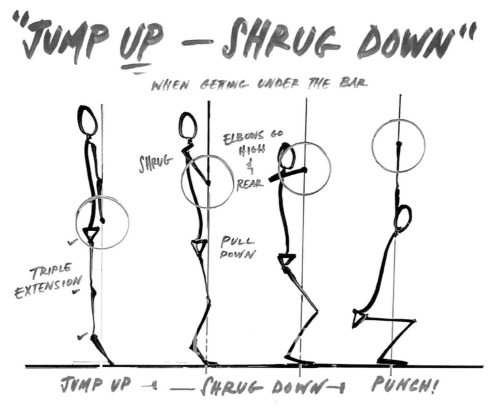

h/t Sage Burgener (@sageburgener)

When?

This cue helps lifters get under the bar in the snatch and clean.

What does this mean?

As the lifter reaches the end of the second pull, there will be full extension through the knees and hip (the jump). The shrug initiates the third pull underneath the bar.

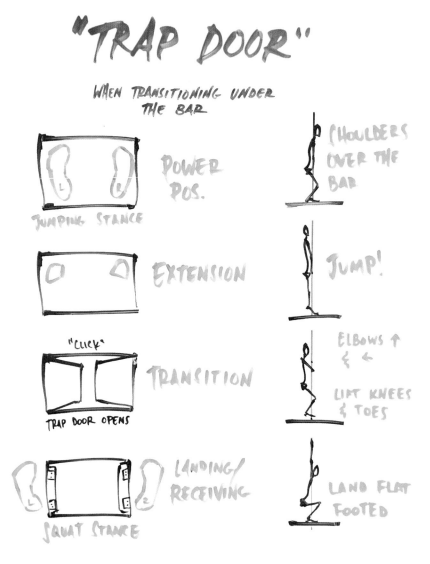

When?

Use this cue to help athletes transition under the bar in the snatch or clean.

What does this mean?

The athlete should imagine they're standing on a trap door. As soon as they jump, it opens, and they must position their feet on either side of it (in a squat stance—landing/receiving position) to avoid falling in!

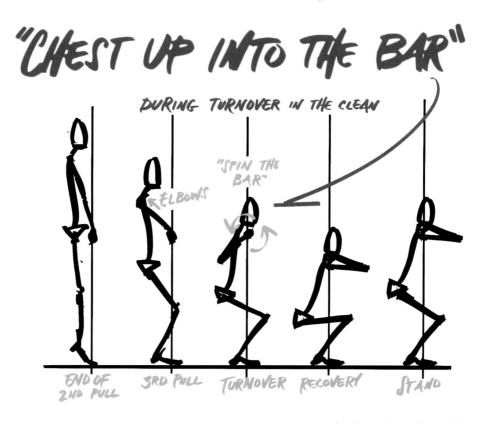

"CHEST UP INTO THE BAR"

DURING TURNOVER IN THE CLEAN

"SPIN THE BAR"

"ELBOWS"

END OF 2ND PULL | 3RD PULL | TURNOVER | RECOVERY | STAND

h/t Greg Everett (@catalystathletics)

When?

Use this cue to describe the turnover in the clean.

What does this mean?

Driving the "chest up into the bar" helps keep the body close to meet the bar smoothly. It also reinforces upright posture to be in the optimal receiving position.

📢 COACHING CUE

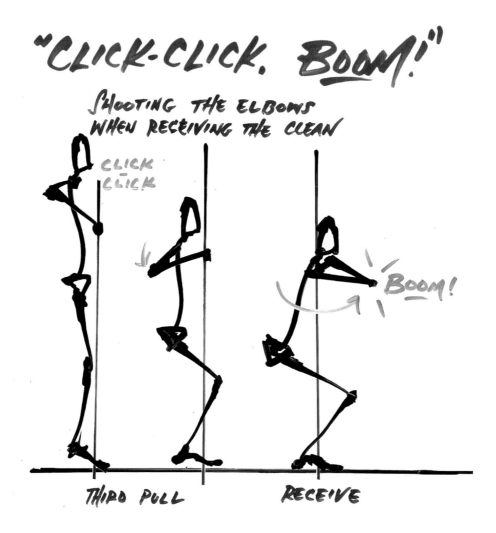

"CLICK-CLICK. BOOM!"

Shooting the elbows when receiving the clean

CLICK CLICK

BOOM!

THIRD PULL

RECEIVE

When?

This cue helps athletes quickly get the elbows around during the receive of the clean.

What does this mean?

This cue is a form of onomatopoeia as it represents the "clicking" of the elbows driving high and back and the *boom* of how fast they must swing around to receive the bar in the front rack position.

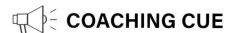

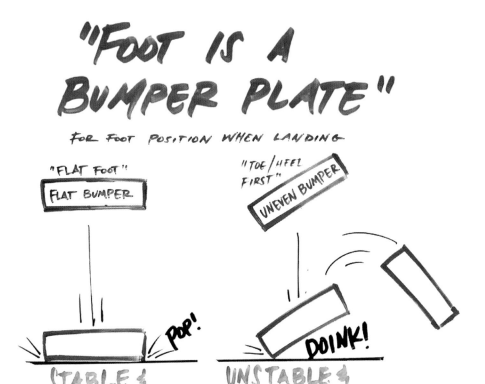

h/t Oleksiy Torokhtiy (@torokhtiy)

When?

Use this cue to describe the foot position when landing during the receive of the clean or snatch.

What does this mean?

When the athlete lands with a full foot, the receive is stable from the ground up—similar to a bumper plate that hits the floor flat.

When the athlete lands toes or heels first, the result is instability from the ground up—similar to a bumper plate that hits the floor on its edge.

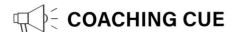

COACHING CUE

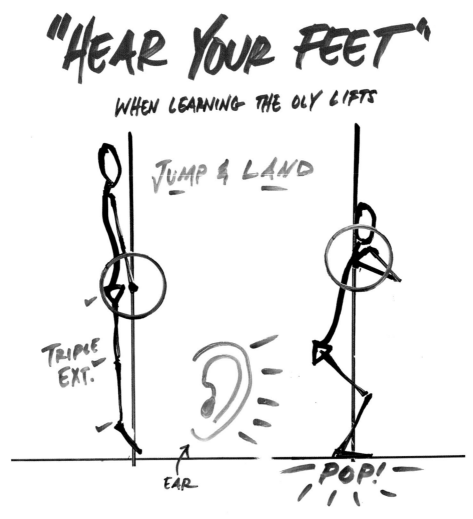

"HEAR YOUR FEET"

WHEN LEARNING THE OLY LIFTS

JUMP & LAND

TRIPLE EXT.

EAR

POP!

h/t Glenn Pendlay (@glenn_pendlay)

When?

This cue is appropriate for athletes who are learning the Olympic lifts.

What does this mean?

During a well-executed lift, the feet transition from a pulling stance in the first and second pulls to a squat stance in the receive. If the feet are quiet, they likely didn't move.

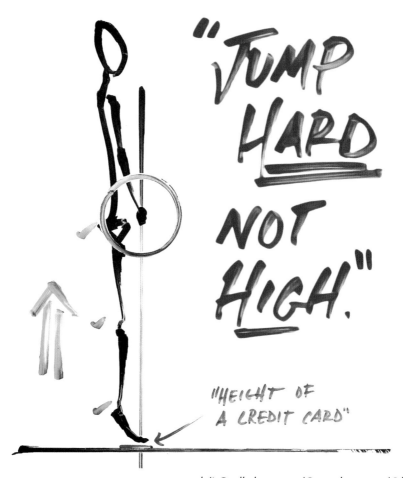

"JUMP HARD NOT HIGH."

"HEIGHT OF A CREDIT CARD"

h/t @mikeburgener/@sageburgener/@burgenerstrength

When?

This cue describes the extension through the second pull of the clean and snatch.

What does this mean?

The extension of the second pull is an explosive jump. However, the split second the bar is weightless, the lifter needs to pull down under the bar rather than going high as for a normal jump.

📢 COACHING CUE

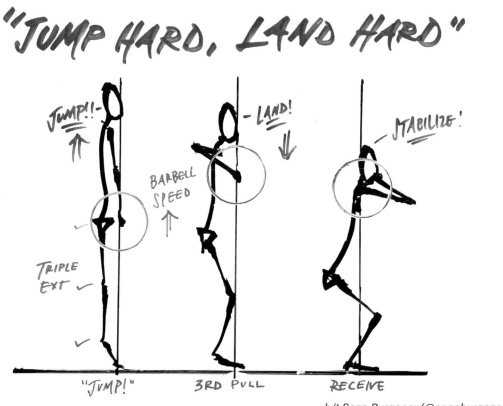

"JUMP HARD, LAND HARD"

JUMP!!

BARBELL SPEED

TRIPLE EXT

LAND!

STABILIZE!

"JUMP!"   3RD PULL   RECEIVE

h/t Sage Burgener (@sageburgener)

When?

This cue describes the transition to receiving during the clean and snatch.

What does this mean?

Immediately after the extension of the second pull, the lifter needs to pull under the bar and into position to receive the bar. This movement must be aggressive to stabilize the lifter's body and the weight.

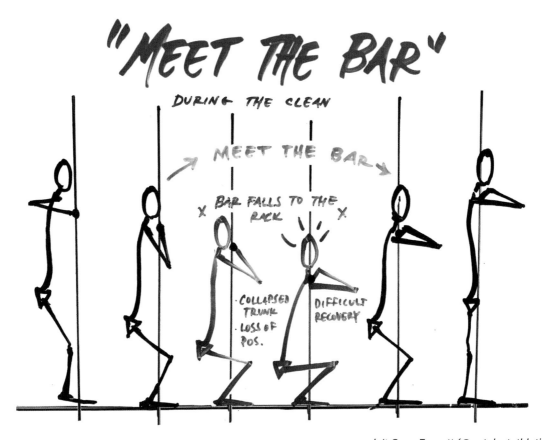

h/t Greg Everett (@catalystathletics)

When?

Use this cue to describe receiving the bar in the clean.

What does this mean?

The goal of the receive is to bring the bar to the shoulders as smoothly as possible. To "meet the bar" simply means meeting the bar at whatever height it's being pulled to.

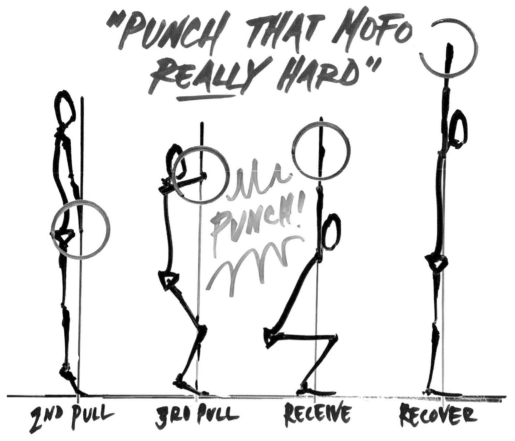

"PUNCH THAT MOFO REALLY HARD"

2ND PULL — 3RD PULL — RECEIVE — RECOVER

h/t Mike Burgener (@mikeburgener)

When?

Use this cue to describe how to receive the bar in a strong position during the snatch.

What does this mean?

Receiving the bar during the snatch needs to be as aggressive as a punch.

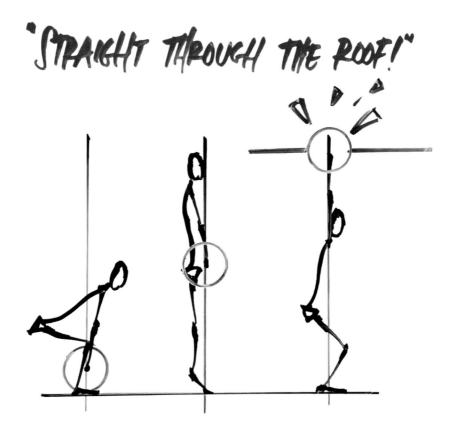

"STRAIGHT THROUGH THE ROOF!"

What does this mean?

As athletes become more proficient in the Olympic lifts, coaches need to get better at teaching them the finer details. Helping them understand how to receive the barbell with strong and active shoulders is imperative.

We often hear, "punch," which is a great cue, but next time try "straight through the roof" to see if it helps the athlete land with a solid upper body.

SPACE

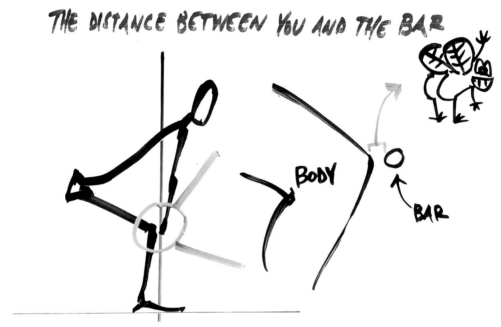

"A GNAT'S ASS"

THE DISTANCE BETWEEN YOU AND THE BAR

BODY

BAR

h/t Sage Burgener (@sageburgener) during the
@burgenerstrength Level 1 Certification

What does this mean?

During a clean or snatch, the space between the bar and the body needs to be as minimal as possible—as close as a "gnat's ass."

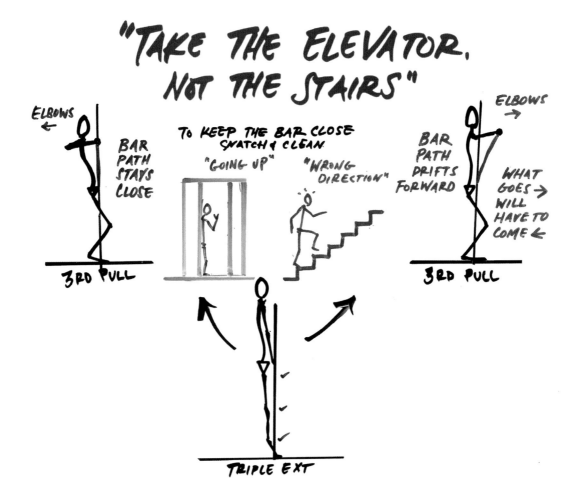

"TAKE THE ELEVATOR, NOT THE STAIRS"

ELBOWS ←
BAR PATH STAYS CLOSE
3RD PULL

TO KEEP THE BAR CLOSE
SNATCH & CLEAN
"GOING UP"
"WRONG DIRECTION"

BAR PATH DRIFTS FORWARD
ELBOWS →
WHAT GOES → WILL HAVE TO COME ←
3RD PULL

TRIPLE EXT

What does this mean?

Generally speaking, the bar should remain as close to the body as possible during the snatch and clean. The visual of the bar taking the path of the elevator (moving vertically) instead of the stairs (moving vertically but also away) may help the athlete understand how to improve their movement.

📢 COACHING CUE

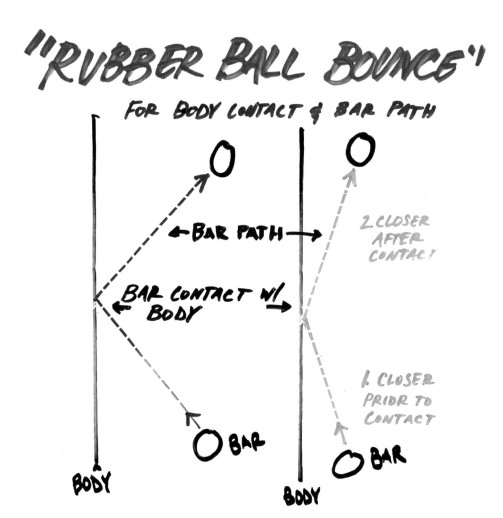

"RUBBER BALL BOUNCE"
FOR BODY CONTACT & BAR PATH

← BAR PATH →

BAR CONTACT w/ BODY

2 CLOSER AFTER CONTACT

1 CLOSER PRIOR TO CONTACT

BODY

BAR

BODY

BAR

h/t Greg Everett (@catalystathletics)

When?

Use this cue to teach bar contact during the Olympic lifts.

What does this mean?

During the pull of the clean and snatch, the bar contacts the body (hips for the snatch, upper thighs for the clean). Prior to contact, the bar should be as close to the body as possible without dragging. Similar to the way a ball bounces against a flat surface, the closer the bar is to the body prior to contact, the closer it will stay after contact.

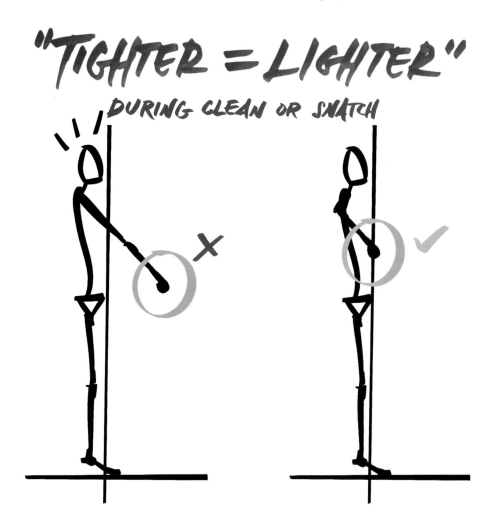

"TIGHTER = LIGHTER"
DURING CLEAN OR SNATCH

What does this mean?

The farther the bar is from the midline of the body, the heavier the bar will feel.

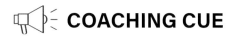

SEQUENCING

"ROCKET FUEL STAGES"

TO DESCRIBE THE SEQUENCE OF
THE SNATCH OR CLEAN

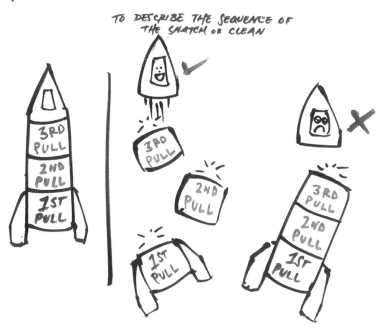

h/t Oleksiy Torokhtiy (@torokhtiy/@torwod)

When?

This cue describes the sequence of pulls during the snatch or clean.

What does this mean?

Just as the snatch or clean has three pulls (first, second, third), a rocket has three fuel stages to drive it into orbit. If a stage engages out of sequence, the rocket will fail. Similarly, if an Olympic lifter engages a pull out of sequence, they will not maximize their power.

Note: This cue also works with rowing: three stages of the drive (legs, back/hips, arms).

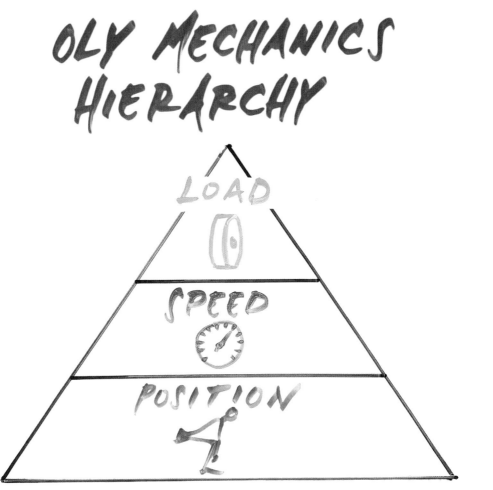

h/t Wil Fleming (@wilfleming)

What does this mean?

First focus on establishing proper positioning by moving slowly and with light weight.

Once the athlete shows consistency with proper positioning, they're ready to add some speed to the movement.

Lastly, the athlete adds load. So, in the final stage, they have good positions, done quickly and with a lot of weight.

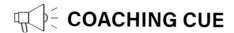

COACHING CUE

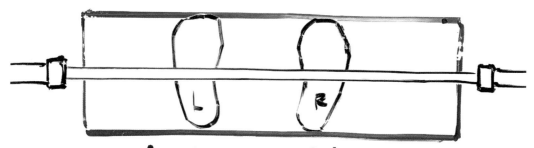

"THE AREA OF THE BASE"

FOR BAR PATH ON OLYMPIC LIFTS

SNATCH OR C&J
THE BAR SHOULD NEVER MOVE
OUTSIDE THE AREA OF THE BASE.

h/t Mike Burgener (@mikeburgener)

When?

This cue describes the bar path for Olympic lifts.

What does this mean?

The area of the base is a rectangular box around the feet that starts with the toes and ends with the heels. Throughout the entire lift of the clean, jerk, and snatch, the bar path should not go outside the area of the base.

CHAPTER ⑤

KETTLEBELL

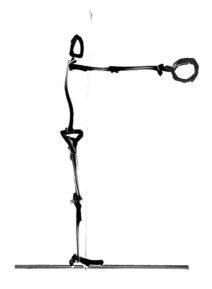

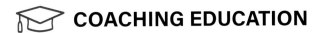

ANATOMY OF A KETTLEBELL

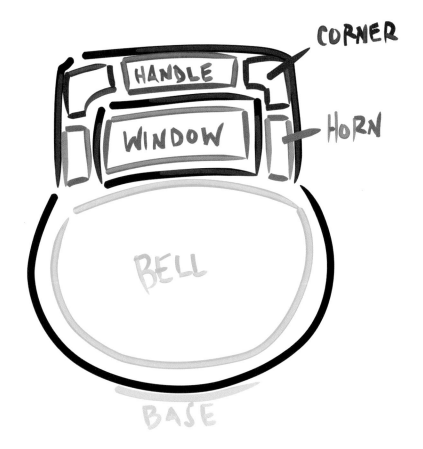

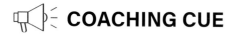
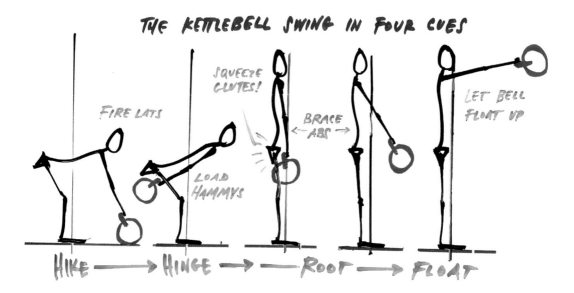

What does this mean?

The kettlebell swing has four distinct phases, which you can explain to athletes with these four cues:

- HIKE the kettlebell back between the legs.
- HINGE the hips back and keep the shins vertical.
- ROOT the feet down into the earth.
- FLOAT the kettlebell up. Don't "muscle" it up with the arms.

"HIKE" THE KETTLEBELL

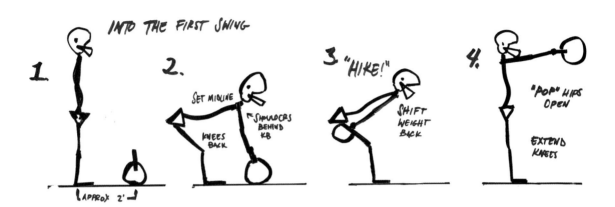

INTO THE FIRST SWING

1

(APPROX 2')

2. SET MIDLINE
SHOULDERS BEHIND KB
KNEES BACK

3 "HIKE!"
SHIFT WEIGHT BACK

4. "POP" HIPS OPEN
EXTEND KNEES

When?

Use this cue to describe getting the kettlebell off the ground and into the first swing.

What does this mean?

1. The athlete should start with the kettlebell approximately 2 feet in front of them (distance will vary depending on the athlete's build).

2. The athlete hinges at the hip, the knees go back, the athlete grabs the KB with their shoulders behind the handle, and they set the midline.

3. The athlete maintains a strong midline, shifts their weight back, and hikes the kettlebell between the legs.

4. The athlete "pops" the hips open and extends the knees.

Why?

Following these steps sets the athlete in a strong position from the very beginning, and it's a more efficient use of energy than deadlifting the kettlebell and getting the swing moving from a dead stop.

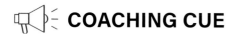

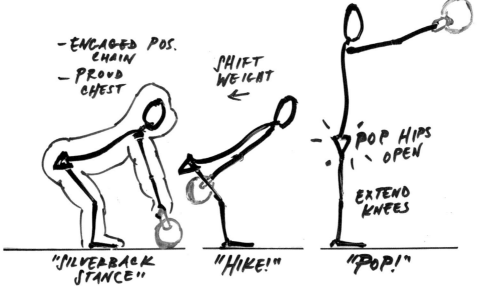

h/t Eugen Loki (@pheasyque) and @phase6fitness

When?

Use this cue to help athletes set up for the kettlebell swing.

What does this mean?

When setting up for the kettlebell swing, the athlete can imagine being a strong silverback gorilla with their chest up and the posterior chain muscles engaged.

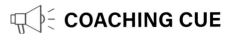

"BE THE ARROW, NOT THE BOW."

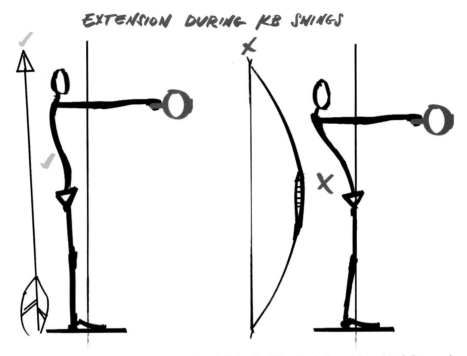

EXTENSION DURING KB SWINGS

h/t Sally Tudor (@saltudor) and Cory Mark (@coachcorymark)

When?

This cue applies to the extension during kettlebell swings to correct the common error of hyperextending the spine during the hip extension.

What does this mean?

This simple phrase may help your athlete avoid hyperextending the spine by imagining their body is a straight arrow, not a curved bow.

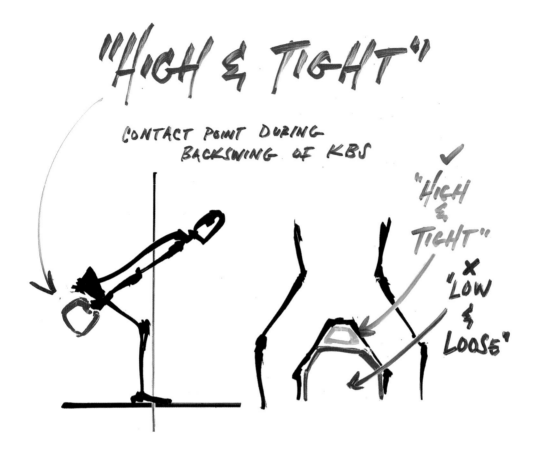

"HIGH & TIGHT"

CONTACT POINT DURING
BACKSWING OF KBS

✓ "HIGH & TIGHT"

✗ "LOW & LOOSE"

When?

Use this cue to describe the contact point during the backswing of the kettlebell swing.

What does this mean?

There should be minimal space between the top of the kettlebell and the athlete's crotch.

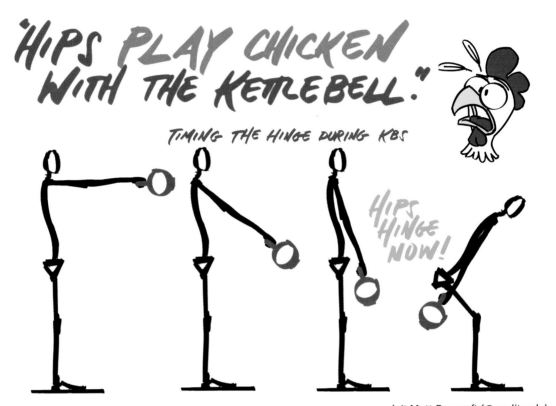

"HIPS PLAY CHICKEN WITH THE KETTLEBELL."

TIMING THE HINGE DURING KBS

HIPS HINGE NOW!

h/t Matt Beecroft (@realitysdc)

When?

This cue describes the timing of the hip hinge of the kettlebell swing.

What does this mean?

During the downswing, allow the kettlebell to come down toward the hips and the elbows to connect to the ribs. At the very last moment, forcefully send the hips back.

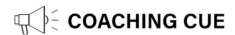

COACHING CUE

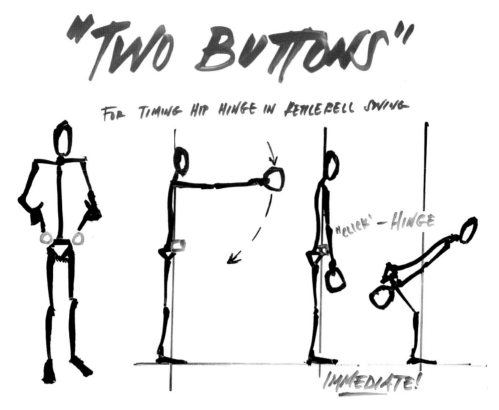

"TWO BUTTONS"

FOR TIMING HIP HINGE IN KETTLEBELL SWING

"CLICK" — HINGE

IMMEDIATE!

h/t Pavel Macek (@pavelmacekcom)/@StrongFirst

When?

This cue addresses the timing for the hip hinge in the kettlebell swing.

What does this mean?

Imagine there are two buttons on either side of the hip points. They switch *on* as soon as the forearms touch them and send the hips into the hinge.

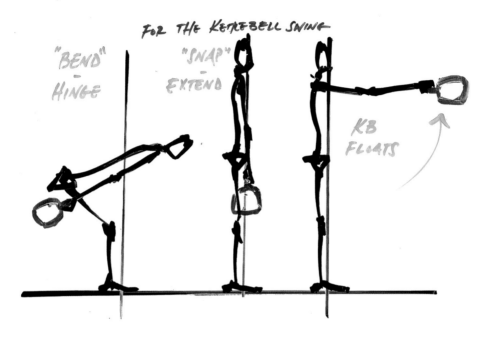

"THE BEND AND SNAP"

FOR THE KETTLEBELL SWING

"BEND" - HINGE

"SNAP" - EXTEND

KB FLOATS

h/t Reese Witherspoon in Legally Blonde

What does this mean?

Although the movement sequence of "The Bend and Snap" from the movie *Legally Blonde* may differ completely from this kettlebell swing movement, the phrase can still be applied:

- **Bend:** The hips hinge back, the knees are slightly bent, and the shins stay vertical.
- **Snap:** The hips and knees aggressively extend, the heels stay grounded, and the athlete stands tall.

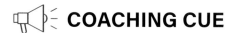

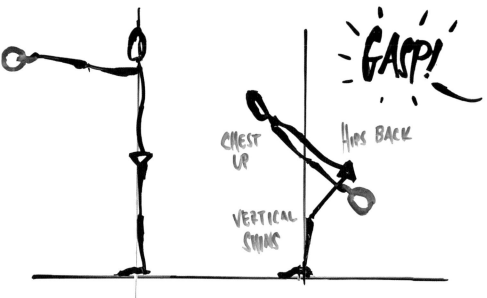

h/t Michael Wille (@michael_wille_)

When?

This cue applies to movements where the athlete is performing a hinge (e.g., good mornings, kettlebell swings, setting up for a clean or snatch).

What does this mean?

This cue may help your athlete understand how to send their hips back and maintain the lumbar curve during the hinge rather than sinking the hips down and rounding the back.

"When performing a hinge, be like Randy Moss and push your hips back and taunt all the Lambeau faithful as you moon the crowd."

—**MICHAEL WILLE** (@michael_wille_)

"DRINKING BIRD"
FOR HIP HINGE MOVEMENTS

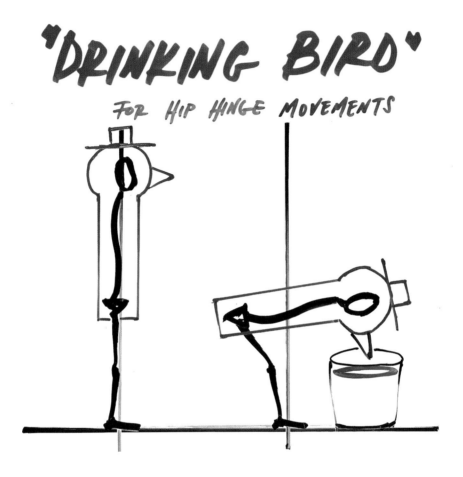

When?

This cue applies to movements that involve performing a hinge (e.g., good mornings, kettlebell swings, setting up for a clean or snatch).

What does this mean?

Throughout the hip hinge movement, the spine should be held in a neutral position. The movement looks similar to the side view of a drinking bird toy. There should be as little deviation from neutral in the lumbar, thoracic, and cervical sections of the spine as possible.

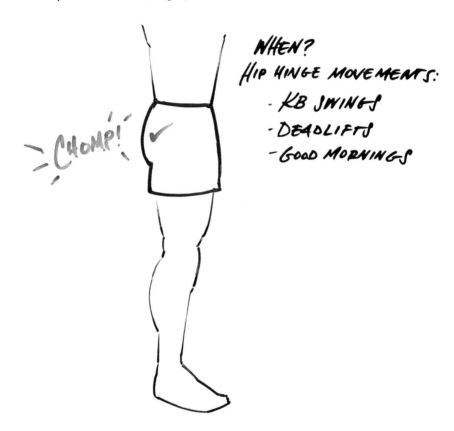

"HUNGRY BUTT"
FOR GLUTE ENGAGEMENT

CHOMP!

WHEN?
HIP HINGE MOVEMENTS:
- KB SWINGS
- DEADLIFTS
- GOOD MORNINGS

When?

Use this to cue glute engagement during hip hinge movements.

What does this mean?

During the hip hinge, the glutes engage to snap the hips forward. This cue may help communicate that "snappiness," as if the butt cheeks are "chomping" the seat of the athlete's shorts.

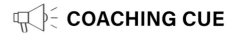
"WET TOWEL SNAP TO THE REAR"

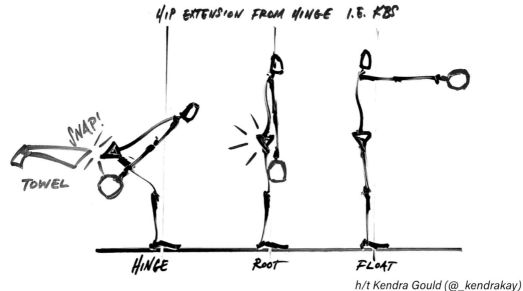

HIP EXTENSION FROM HINGE I.E. KBS

SNAP!

TOWEL

HINGE   ROOT   FLOAT

h/t Kendra Gould (@_kendrakay)

When?

This cue describes the powerful opening of the hip hinge.

What does this mean?

The extension of the hip hinge should be powerful, similar to the reaction one has after being snapped in the rear end with a wet towel.

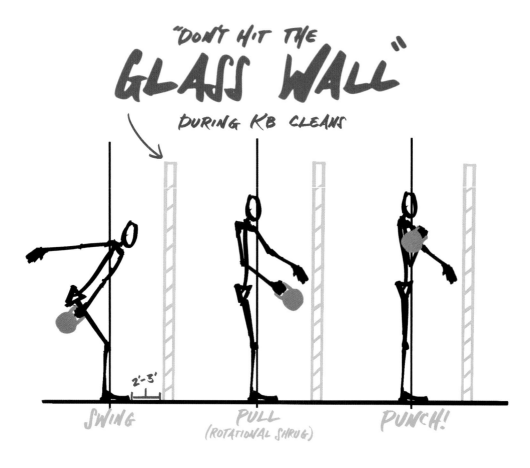

"DON'T HIT THE
GLASS WALL"
DURING KB CLEANS

SWING | PULL (ROTATIONAL SHRUG) | PUNCH!

2'-3'

When?

This cue applies to the kettlebell clean.

What does this mean?

The athlete should imagine they are standing 2 to 3 feet behind a glass wall, and they want to avoid having the kettlebell crash into it. This concept helps encourage the athlete to keep the trajectory of the swing close to the body.

Why?

A common error during the kettlebell clean is allowing the upper portion of the active arm to detach from the torso. When that happens, the kettlebell swings forward, which is less efficient and ultimately causes the kettlebell to crash back into the athlete.

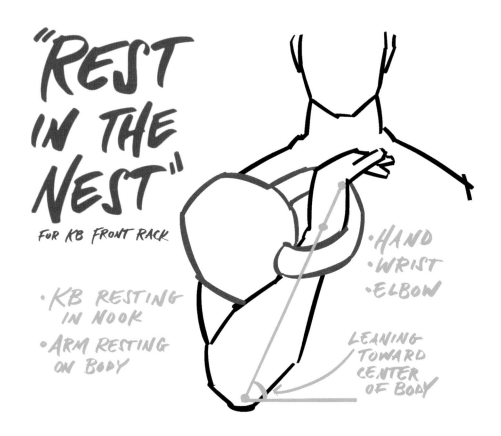

"REST IN THE NEST"

FOR KB FRONT RACK

- KB RESTING IN NOOK
- ARM RESTING ON BODY

- HAND
- WRIST
- ELBOW

LEANING TOWARD CENTER OF BODY

When?

This cue describes the kettlebell front rack.

What does this mean?

During the kettlebell front rack, the bell rests in the nest (nook) of the supporting arm. The arm is resting on the body with the elbow on the crest of the hip. The hand, wrist, and elbow should make a straight line that is leaning toward the centerline of the body.

📢 COACHING CUE

"DIP - DRIVE - PUNCH!"

TO JERK: BARBELL, DUMBBELL, KETTLEBELL

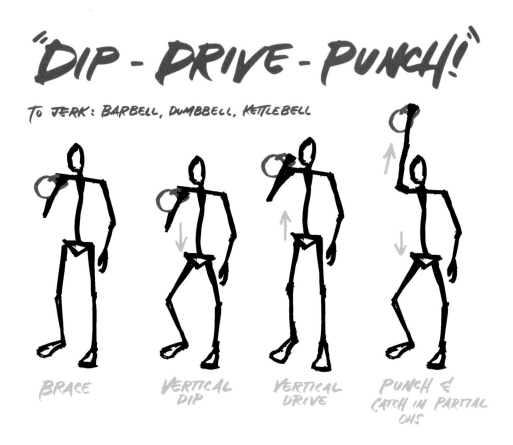

BRACE   VERTICAL DIP   VERTICAL DRIVE   PUNCH & CATCH IN PARTIAL OHS

What does this mean?

This simple three-word phrase helps communicate the sequence for the jerk.

- **Dip:** Vertical dip with the knees flexed and tracking over the toes and the shoulders-hips-ankles line straight.

- **Drive:** Vertical drive when the hips and knees extend rapidly and the shoulders-hips-ankles line remains straight.

- **Punch:** The momentum from the drive carries into a punch overhead as the athlete catches the kettlebell in a partial overhead squat.

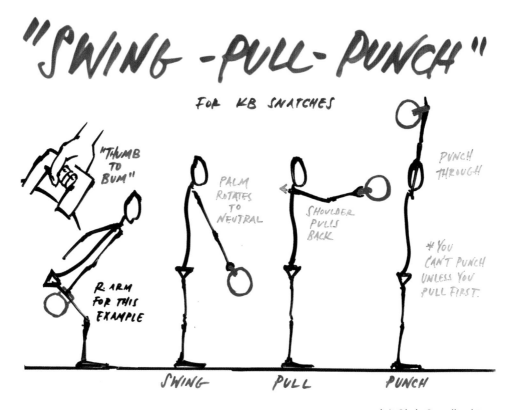

h/t Chris Spealler (@cspealler)

What does this mean?

This simple three-word phrase helps communicate the mechanics of the kettlebell snatch.

- **Swing:** The athlete should start with a swing, just to their waist, with their hand going from palm inside to neutral.

- **Pull:** At the top of the swing, the shoulder is going to come back, which keeps things close to the body.

- **Punch:** Punch through at the end but allow the kettlebell to rotate on top of the hand and wrist.

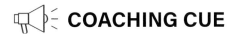
COACHING CUE

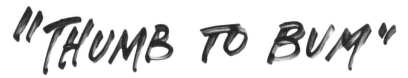

"THUMB TO BUM"

FOR SINGLE ARM KB SWINGS

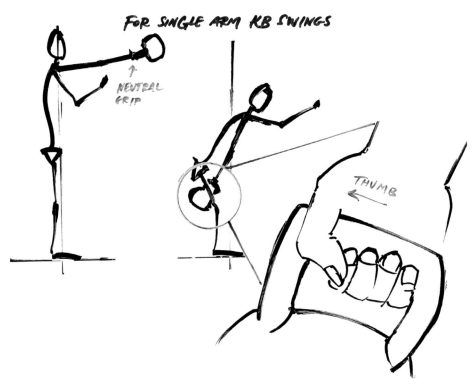

NEUTRAL GRIP

THUMB

h/t Sebastian Jago (coach_sabby_j)

What does this mean?

During the backswing of a single-arm kettlebell swing, the athlete allows the bell to rotate from a neutral position so the thumb is pointed backward.

Why?

The turn from the neutral position to pointing the thumb backward helps the athlete generate more torque and power.

THE KETTLEBELL WINDMILL

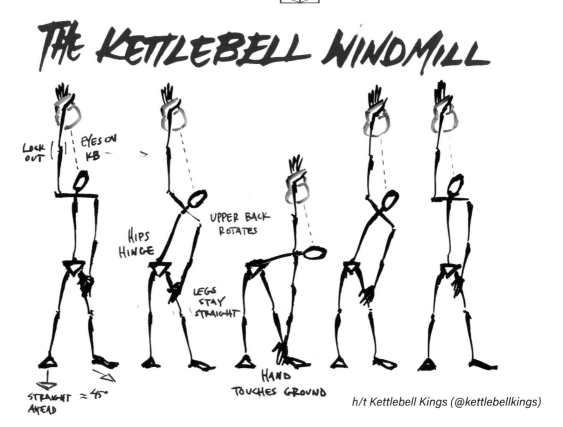

LOCK OUT | EYES ON KB

HIPS HINGE

UPPER BACK ROTATES

LEGS STAY STRAIGHT

HAND TOUCHES GROUND

STRAIGHT AHEAD ≈ 45°

h/t Kettlebell Kings (@kettlebellkings)

Points of performance

- The kettlebell is extended overhead with one arm.

- The foot on the same side as the kettlebell is facing forward.

- The other foot is turned out at approximately a 45° angle.

- The more narrow the stance, the more mobility is needed.

- The free hand is placed on the inside of the thigh.

- The athlete should look up at kettlebell, keeping eyes on it throughout the movement.

- The athlete hinges their hips at a slight angle opposite the unloaded side.

- The upper back rotates throughout the descent.

- The knees stay fully extended.

- The free hand reaches for the ground by following the inside of the leg.

- Once the hand touches the ground, the athlete reverses the movements to the starting position.

Note: Scale the movement by widening the stance and/or moving partially through the ROM.

📢 COACHING CUE

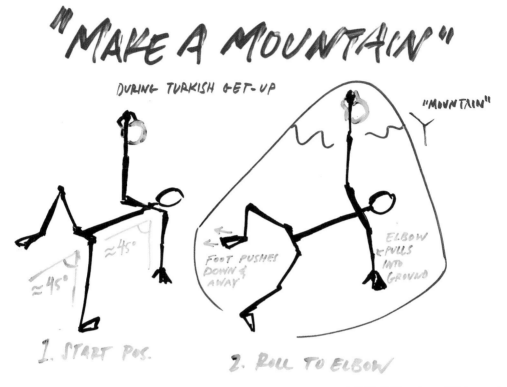

"MAKE A MOUNTAIN"

DURING TURKISH GET-UP

"MOUNTAIN"

≈45°

≈45°

FOOT PUSHES DOWN & AWAY

ELBOW PULLS INTO GROUND

1. START POS.

2. ROLL TO ELBOW

h/t Matt Kingstone (@king_cobra_fit)

When?

This cue describes the roll to the elbow during the Turkish get-up.

What does this mean?

Imagine that the foot on the floor of the bell side is one land mass and the elbow on the floor is another. Drive these two land masses together to raise the bell toward the sky.

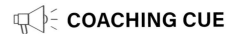
"USE YOUR THUMB AS A SIGHT."

DURING THE TURKISH GET-UP

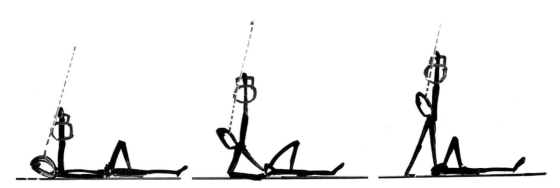

h/t Jeff Martone (@jeffmartone)

When?

Use this cue to explain how to move between the arm-extension step and the sit-up step of the Turkish get-up.

What does this mean?

To keep their arm straight during the Turkish get-up, the athlete can sight along their arm to the thumb.

> *"Wherever my thumb is, I sight it like a firearm; where it is on the ceiling, that's where it stays."*

—**JEFF MARTONE,** founder and CEO of @TacitcalAthlete_TS

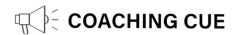
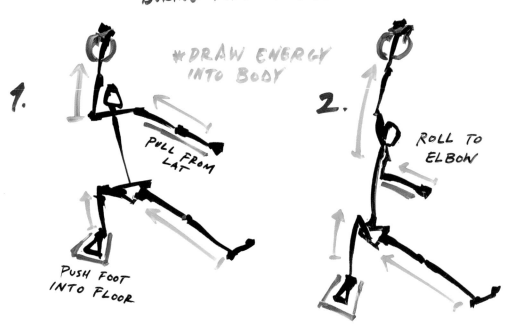

Green lines show energy flowing into the body.

Orange lines show where force is applied to initiate the movement.

When?

This cue applies to the Turkish get-up.

What does this mean?

The key to the Turkish get-up is understanding the energy flow and tension, especially during the "roll to elbow." The athlete *pushes* the floor with the foot and *pulls* the lat of the non-bell arm. This helps them roll to the elbow.

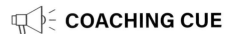
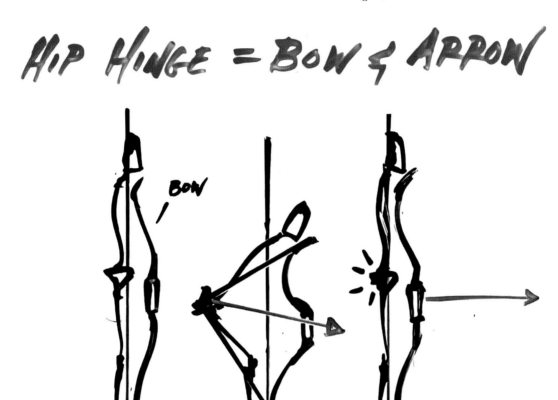

What does this mean?

Imagine the hips are the string of a bow and the head and feet are the tips of the bow. As the hips go back, the string stretches. The "bow" between the head and feet snaps the hips forward.

CHAPTER 6

RUNNING/ SPRINTING

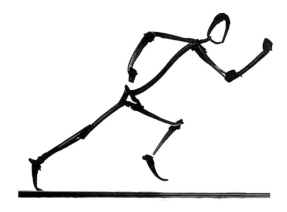

"HUMAN BODY IS A WHEEL"

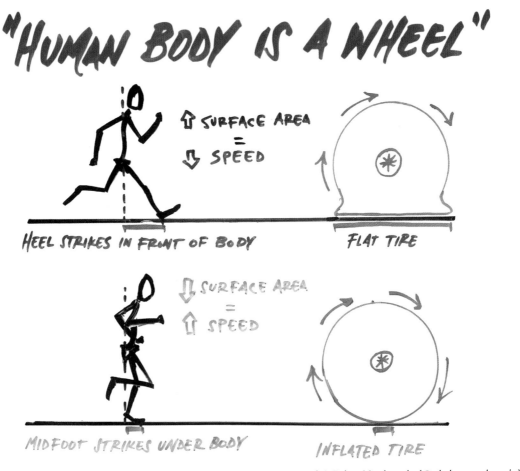

⬆ SURFACE AREA
=
⬇ SPEED

HEEL STRIKES IN FRONT OF BODY

FLAT TIRE

⬇ SURFACE AREA
=
⬆ SPEED

MIDFOOT STRIKES UNDER BODY

INFLATED TIRE

h/t Brian Mackenzie (@_brianmackenzie)

When?

Use this cue to teach athletes to keep the foot strike underneath the body and pull the heel up to the hip.

What does this mean?

The more contact a runner has with the ground, the slower they are.

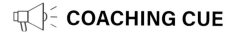

COACHING CUE

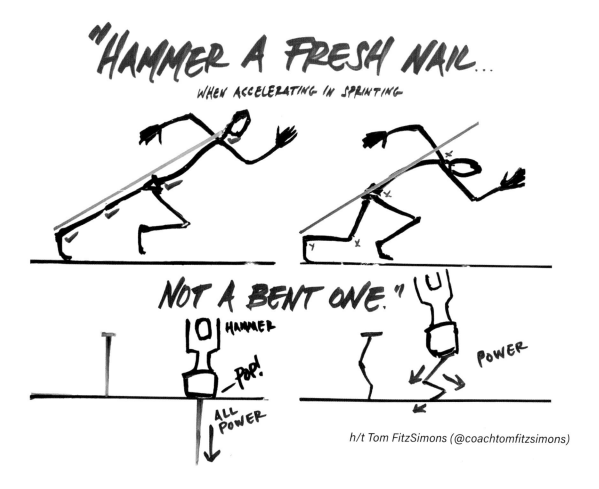

h/t Tom FitzSimons (@coachtomfitzsimons)

When?

This cue describes acceleration in sprinting.

What does this mean?

When applying force into the ground, the body should be in alignment. Runners should avoid breaking at the hips and rounding the back in the shape of a bent nail.

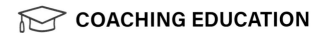

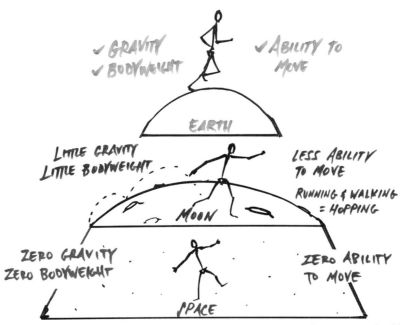

h/t Pose Method (@posemethod)

What does this mean?

Muscles are rendered useless if a person can't apply their bodyweight.

In space, zero gravity = zero bodyweight = zero movement

A person needs some sort of support or interaction with another object to move.

On the moon, little gravity = little bodyweight = little ability to move

Walking/running becomes hopping.

On Earth, gravity = bodyweight = movement

Movement is possible through the application of bodyweight.

Conclusion

To run efficiently, runners need to transfer the downward force of gravity into horizontal movement.

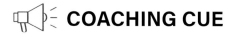
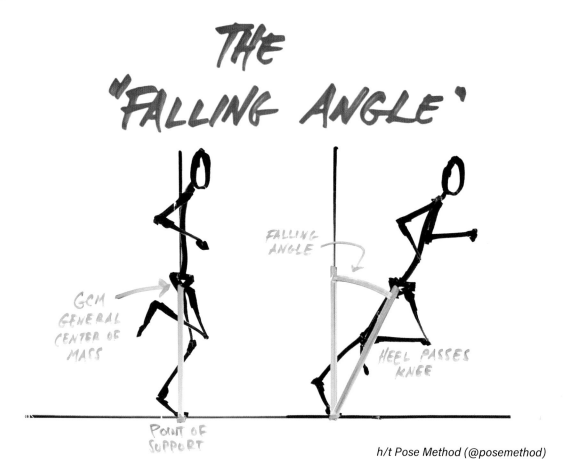

h/t Pose Method (@posemethod)

What does this mean?

The falling angle of the body occurs when the foot of the swing leg passes the knee of the support leg. When the runner allows the body to fall forward, they redirect the force of gravity by rotating around a fixed point.

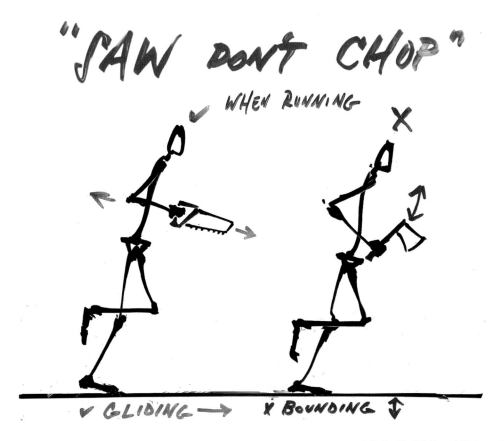

"SAW DON'T CHOP"
WHEN RUNNING

✔ GLIDING → ✗ BOUNDING ↕

h/t Dr. Matt Minard (@learn.2.run)

What does this mean?

To maximize horizontal movement and minimize bouncing when running, imagine the forearms are hand saws. With efficient running, the arms and legs are in synchronization to move the body forward.

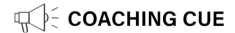
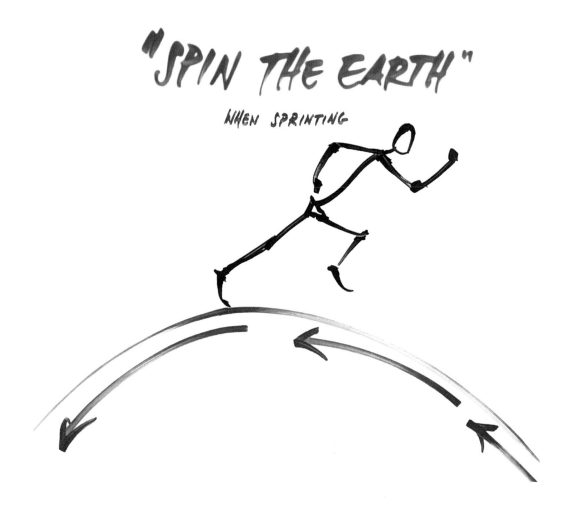

What does this mean?

This cue may help athletes visualize how to optimally produce horizontal force to sprint. It's as if they are leaning forward to spin a giant wheel.

CHAPTER 7

ROWING

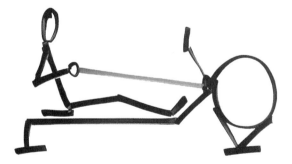

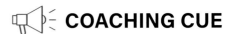

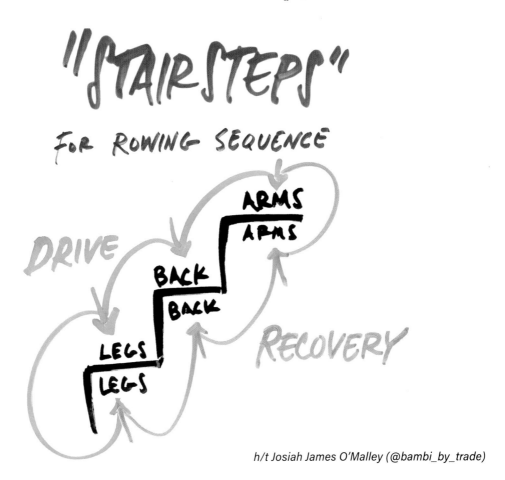

h/t Josiah James O'Malley (@bambi_by_trade)

What does this mean?

The sequence for efficient rowing technique can be described as a set of stairs. The "drive" steps go up, and the "recovery" steps go down. During the drive, the rower starts with the legs, then the back, and finally the arms. During the recovery, the rower moves back down the stairs: arms, back, legs. The overall drive/recovery ratio should be 1:2. In other words, the recovery should take twice as long as the drive.

ROWING SEQUENCE

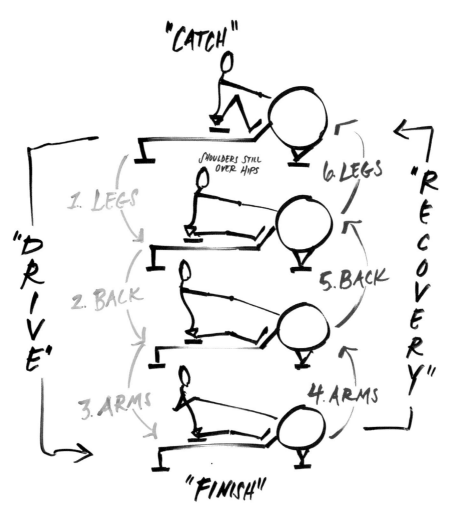

h/t Concept2 (@concept2inc)

Points of performance

The Catch

- The arms are straight, the head is neutral, and the shoulders are level and not hunched.

- The upper body leans forward from the hips with the shoulders in front of the hips.

- The shins are vertical, or as close to vertical as is comfortable. The shins should not move beyond perpendicular.

- The heels may lift as needed.

The Drive

- The rower starts the drive by pressing with the legs and then swinging the back through the vertical position before finally adding the arm pull.

- The hands should move in a straight line to and from the flywheel.

- The shoulders remain low and relaxed.

The Recovery

- The rower extends the arms until they straighten before leaning from the hips toward the flywheel.

- Once the hands have cleared the knees, the knees are allowed to bend and gradually slide the seat forward on the monorail.

- For the next stroke, the rower returns to the catch position with the shoulders relaxed and the shins vertical.

The Finish

- The upper body leans back slightly, with good support from the core muscles.

- The legs are extended, and the handle is held slightly below the ribs.

- The shoulders should be low with the wrists and grip relaxed. The wrists should be flat.

Need more help?

For more information, check out @darkhorserowing.

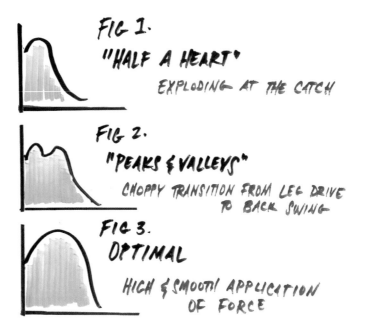

FORCE CURVE — CONCEPT 2 ERG

FIG 1.
"HALF A HEART"
EXPLODING AT THE CATCH

FIG 2.
"PEAKS & VALLEYS"
CHOPPY TRANSITION FROM LEG DRIVE TO BACK SWING

FIG 3.
OPTIMAL
HIGH & SMOOTH APPLICATION OF FORCE

What does this mean?

The smoother the curve, the smoother the application of force. The larger the area under the curve, the greater the amount of force applied.

Figure 1, "Half a heart": Exploding at the catch (applying great force at the beginning of the drive) results in a sharp curve and steep drop.

Figure 2, "Peaks and valleys": The rower is experiencing poor transition of power from the leg drive to the body swing to the arm pull.

Figure 3, "Optimal": The rower is exerting a high and smooth application of force.

Need more information?

To see the force curve while an athlete is rowing, press Change Display on the monitor until the curve displays. For more information, check out "Using the Force Curve" on the Concept2 website.

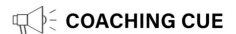
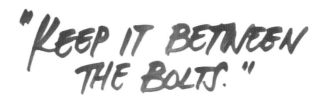

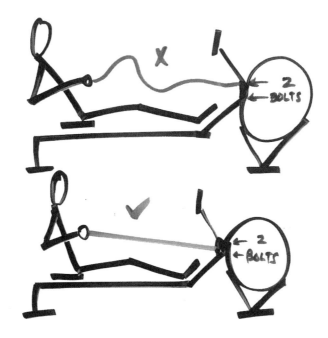

When?

This visual aid helps athletes keep the chain level.

Why?

To maximize efficiency during the rowing stroke, try to keep the chain between the bolts on the Concept2 erg's chain guide.

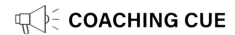
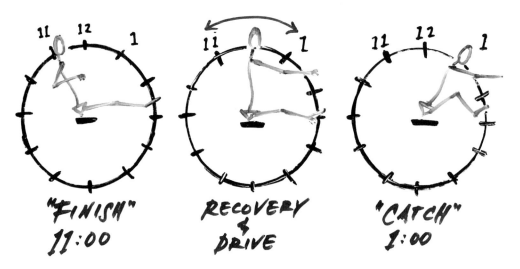

"ROWER'S HAPPY HOUR: SERVED B/N: 11:00 & 1:00"

FOR BACK POSITIONS

"FINISH" 11:00

RECOVERY & DRIVE

"CATCH" 1:00

When?

Use this cue to describe the position of the back during rowing.

What does this mean?

To maximize efficiency while rowing, set the finish position at 11:00 and the catch position at 1:00.

Need more help?

For more information, please see "Common Rowing Technique Errors on Indoor Rowing Machines" by @concept2usa on YouTube.

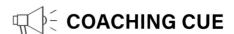
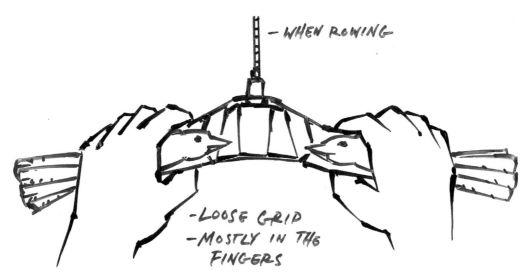

"GRIP THE HANDLE LIKE YOU'RE HOLDING TWO BIRDS."

— WHEN ROWING

- LOOSE GRIP
- MOSTLY IN THE FINGERS

h/t Alicia Clark (@alicia_r_clark) via @ucanrow2

What does this mean?

The athlete needs to have a loose grip on the outer edge of the handle, as if they are holding a bird in each hand. This helps the athlete to use their lats on the drive and have a more comfortable and strong finish.

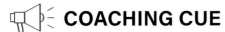
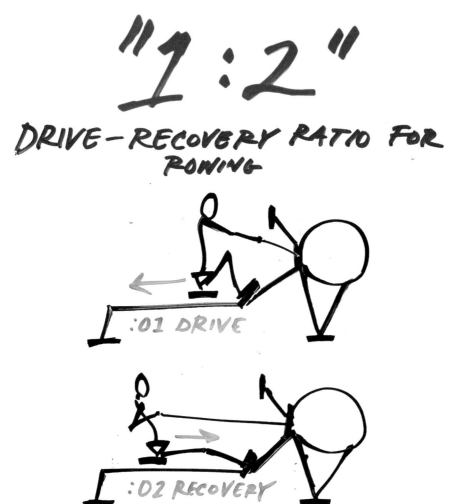

When?

Use this cue to describe the drive-recovery ratio for rowing.

What does this mean?

The recovery should take twice as long as the drive. If the drive is 1 second long, the recovery should be 2 seconds.

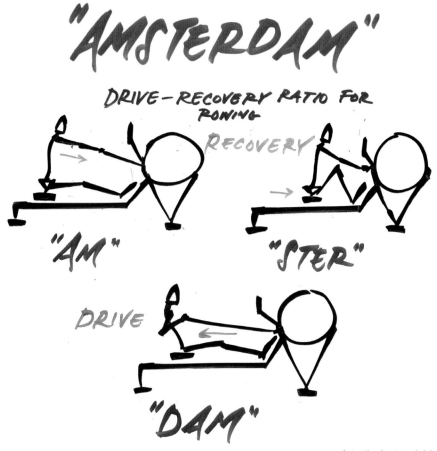

h/t Flavio Garrisi (@flaviogarrisi)

When?

This is another mnemonic device for the drive-recovery ratio during rowing.

What does this mean?

Your recovery should take twice as long as your drive. Imagine saying "Am-ster" (recovery) "dam" (drive).

Here are some other phrases that work:

- "Pine-apple" (recovery) "chunks" (drive)
- "Ham and" (recovery) "cheese" (drive)
- "Fan-tas" (recovery) "tic" (drive)

CHAPTER (8)

MOBILITY

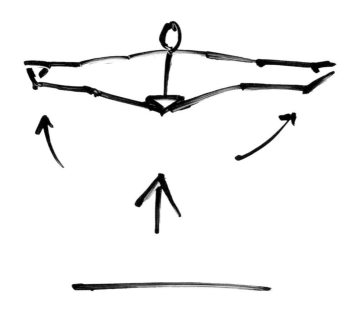

MOBILITY
LEADS TO
BETTER POSITIONING
LEADS TO
MOVEMENT EFFICIENCY
LEADS TO
STRENGTH

What does this mean?

Strength begins with mobility—the ability to take the body through a range of motion with control.

Improving mobility leads to the ability to get into better positioning. Once an athlete can get into a better position, they can build efficiency in moving in and out of that position. After that is established, they can then build strength throughout the range of that movement.

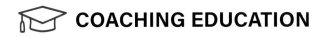
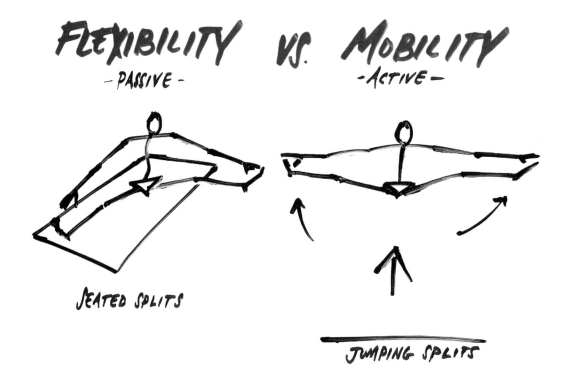

FLEXIBILITY vs. MOBILITY
- PASSIVE - -ACTIVE-

SEATED SPLITS

JUMPING SPLITS

What does this mean?

Flexibility is the ability of a joint to reach full range of motion passively (e.g., seated splits).

Mobility is the active range of motion (e.g., jump splits).

You will never have more mobility than flexibility.

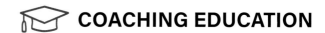

IDENTIFYING A MOVEMENT ISSUE

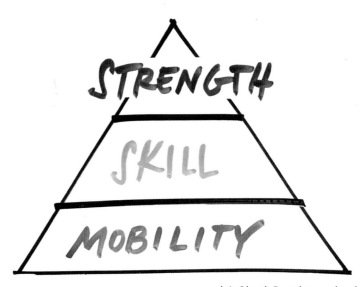

h/t Chuck Bennington (@chuckbennington)

What does this mean?

To help athletes who have trouble performing a specific movement properly, keep the following things in mind:

- **Mobility:** Can the athletes place themselves in the correct position? For example, to determine if athletes can squat to a proper depth (hip crease below the top of the knee), have them try to sit on a box that allows proper depth and positioning. If the athletes can't do that, mobility should be improved before adding load.

- **Skill:** Once mobility has been corrected, athletes need to develop the skill of learning the movement pattern for getting in and out of this position unassisted. As with any skill, this is developed through repetition.

- **Strength:** After mobility and skill have been developed for proper movement, load may be introduced.

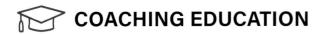
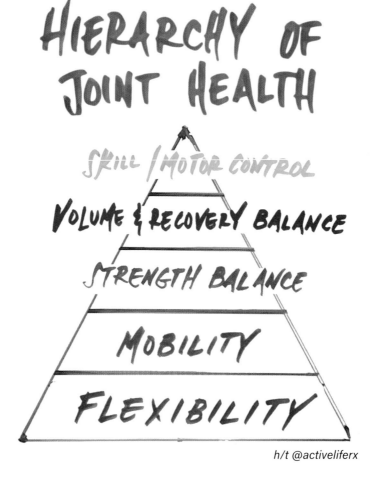

h/t @activeliferx

What does this mean?

Flexibility: The ability of a joint to passively reach a full range of motion.

Mobility: The ability of a joint to actively reach a full range of motion.

Strength balance: The muscles surrounding the joint create an even contraction, and loads are evenly distributed.

Volume and recovery balance: Adequate rest is required to heal and allow for positive adaptation.

Skill/motor control: The athlete who has more flexibility, mobility, and strength balance will be able to more quickly and effectively acquire motor skill.

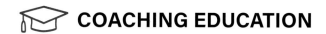

MOVEMENT HIERARCHIES
RELATIVE TO MOBILITY DEMANDS

PULLING
^
CONV. DEADLIFT
SUMO DL
GOOD MORNING
KB SWING
OLYMPIC LIFTS FROM HANG

BILATERAL SQUAT
^
OVERHEAD SQUAT
FRONT SQUAT
HIGH BAR BACK SQ.
LOW BAR BACK SQ.
BOX SQUAT

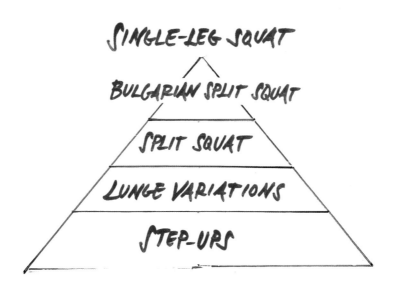

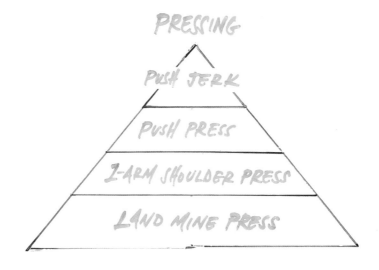

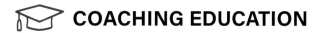

What does this mean?

Pulling Hierarchy Relative to Mobility Demands

- Olympic lifts from the hang
- KB swing
- Good morning, stiff-leg Romanian deadlift, GHD hip extension
- Olympic pull
- Sumo deadlift
- Conventional deadlift

Bilateral Squat Hierarchy Relative to Mobility Demands

- Box squat
- Low bar back squat
- High bar back squat
- Front squat
- Overhead squat

Single-Leg Squat Hierarchy Relative to Mobility Demands

- Step-ups
- Lunge variations
- Split squat
- Bulgarian split squat

Pressing Hierarchy Relative to Mobility Demands

- Land mine press
- One-arm shoulder press
- Barbell shoulder press and push press
- Push jerk and behind-the-neck shoulder press

CHAPTER (9)

BRACING

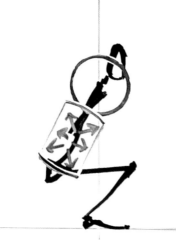

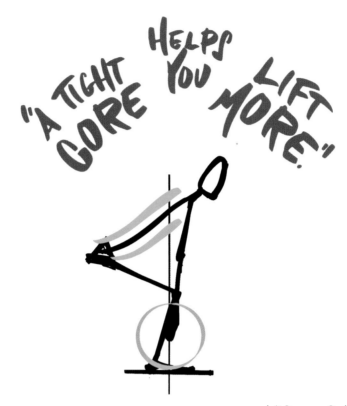

h/t Spencer Smith (@spencergsmith)

When?

This cue applies to lifting anything.

What does this mean?

This simple rhyme may help athletes remember to brace their core and remain tight while lifting anything off the ground.

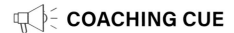
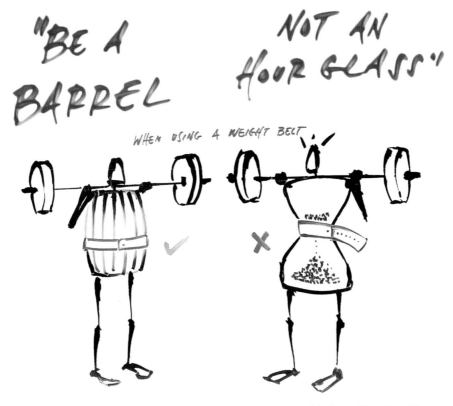

h/t CrossFit G-Steel (@crossfitgsteel)

When?

This cue applies to using a weightlifting belt.

What does this mean?

During a heavy lift, the torso is best supported through a diaphragmatic breath that expands in all directions coupled with a muscular engagement throughout the spine. Wearing a weightlifting belt properly does *not* mean simply cinching it as tight as possible so that the athlete ends up looking like an hourglass.

The athlete should adjust the belt so there is enough room to breathe *into* the belt, allowing it to add another layer of support to the body's natural bracing, similar to a hoop around a barrel.

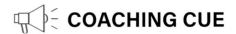
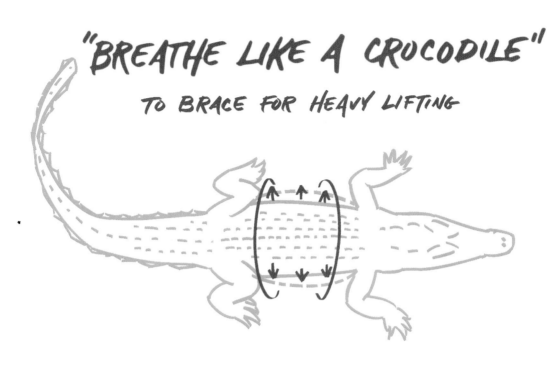

"BREATHE LIKE A CROCODILE"
TO BRACE FOR HEAVY LIFTING

When?

Use this cue to help athletes incorporate diaphragmatic breathing (belly breathing) to brace under load (e.g., heavy squats).

What does this mean?

When a crocodile breathes, its torso expands 360°. When bracing to lift a heavy load, mimicking the crocodile's technique allows the athlete to safely maximize intra-abdominal pressure (IAP) and create a strong stable core.

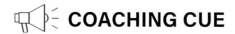 **COACHING CUE**

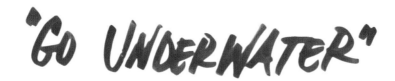

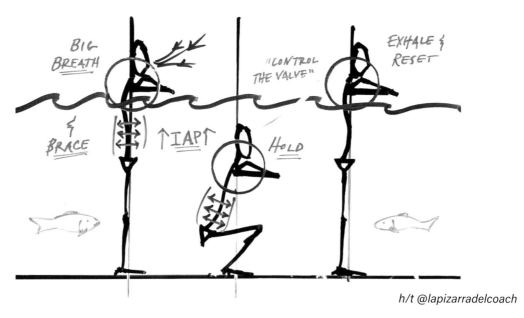

h/t @lapizarradelcoach

When?

This cue teaches breath control during the squat/front squat.

What does this mean?

When squatting heavy weights, it may help the athlete to imagine they are standing in chest-deep water. In that case, they would take a deep breath prior to lowering under the water. Taking a deep breath before squatting helps increase the IAP to stabilize the core.

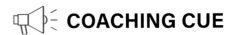

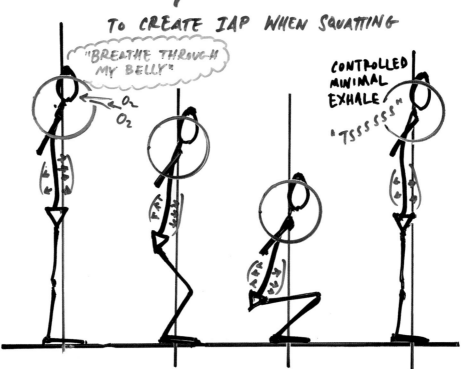

h/t Louie Simmons (@westsidebarbellofficial) via Dave Tate (@underthebar)

When?

Use this cue to help athletes create IAP—the body's "natural weightlifting belt."

What does this mean?

When lifting heavy weight while wearing a weight belt, the athlete should try pushing their belly into the belt as if they are trying to look as fat as possible. Doing so helps increase the intra-abdominal pressure to stabilize the core.

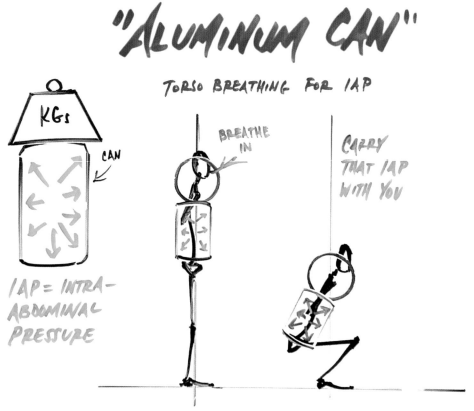

"ALUMINUM CAN"

TORSO BREATHING FOR IAP

KGs

CAN

BREATHE IN

CARRY THAT IAP WITH YOU

IAP = INTRA-ABDOMINAL PRESSURE

h/t Eugen Loki (@pheasyque)

When?

Use this cue to explain how to create IAP when under load.

What does this mean?

When an athlete breathes in and braces, they are pushing air into their lungs and pushing down the diaphragm. This contracts and creates pressure—similar to the pressure in the rigid cylinder of an unopened aluminum can—over the abdominal cavity, obliques, and lumbar muscles.

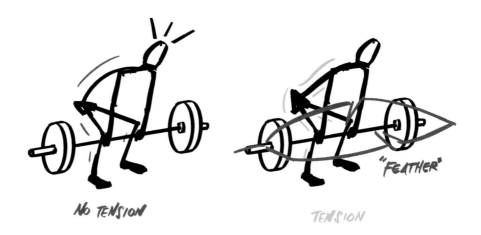

"TIGHTER = LIGHTER"

BODY TENSION CREATES POWER & STABILITY

NO TENSION   TENSION   "FEATHER"

What does this mean?

Use body tension to create power and stability during weightlifting and ultimately to make the weight feel lighter.

CHAPTER (10)

GRIP

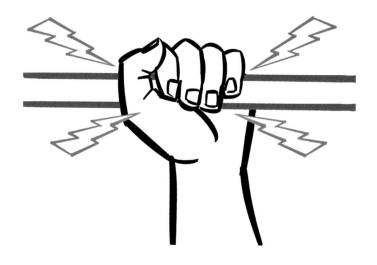

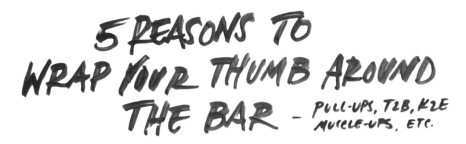

5 REASONS TO WRAP YOUR THUMB AROUND THE BAR

— PULL-UPS, T2B, K2E MUSCLE-UPS, ETC.

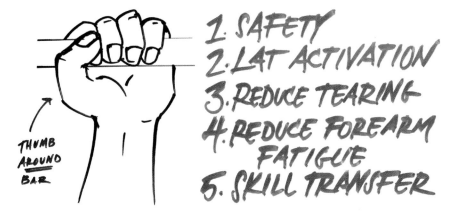

THUMB AROUND BAR

1. SAFETY
2. LAT ACTIVATION
3. REDUCE TEARING
4. REDUCE FOREARM FATIGUE
5. SKILL TRANSFER

What does this mean?

1. **Safety:** Wrapped thumbs act as a safety lock, helping to prevent the hands from slipping.

2. **Lat activation:** Wrapped thumbs allow for better torque on the bar (especially during bar muscle-ups) through more efficient lat activation.

3. **Reduces tearing:** Wrapped thumbs place the hands in a more efficient position to avoid ripping calluses.

4. **Reduces forearm fatigue:** Wrapped thumbs allow for activation through the lats rather than the forearms.

5. **Skill transfer:** Gripping with the thumb translates to the grip on a kettlebell, barbell, or rope.

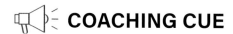
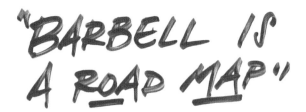

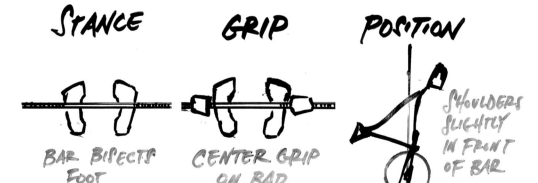

When?

This cue applies to setting stance, grip, and position for a barbell lift.

What does this mean?

Similar to a road map, the barbell can direct the athlete where to go when setting stance, grip, and position for a lift. Here's an example for the deadlift:

- **Stance:** The athlete stands at the center of the bar, according to the knurling marks. The bar bisects the feet in half from a top-down view.

- **Grip:** The grip is evenly centered according to the knurling marks.

- **Position:** The shoulders are slightly in front of the bar.

Note: These positions are general approximations. Everyone is different.

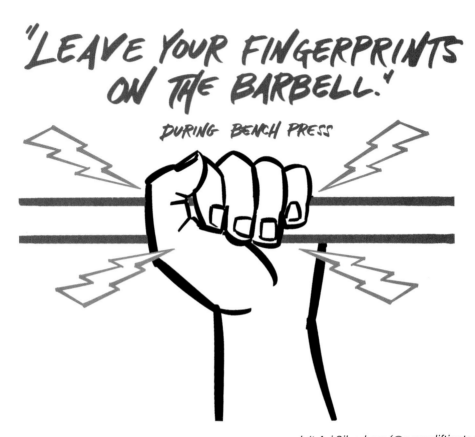

"LEAVE YOUR FINGERPRINTS ON THE BARBELL."

DURING BENCH PRESS

h/t Avi Silverberg (@powerliftingtechnique)

When?

Use this cue for coaching the bench press.

What does this mean?

The hands and arms are packed with muscles, so be sure to use them. A tighter grip on the bar provides more control, which is a major benefit for the bench press.

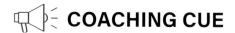

"GRIP THE GROUND"

FOR PUSH-UPS AND HSPUs

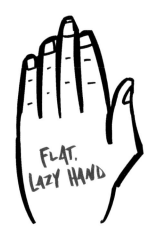

FLAT, LAZY HAND

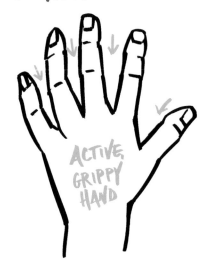

ACTIVE, GRIPPY HAND

When?

This cue applies to push-ups and handstand push-ups.

What does this mean?

When performing push-ups and handstand push-ups, the athlete should recruit as much from the upper body as possible. Torque is created by externally rotating through the shoulders and arms by gripping the ground.

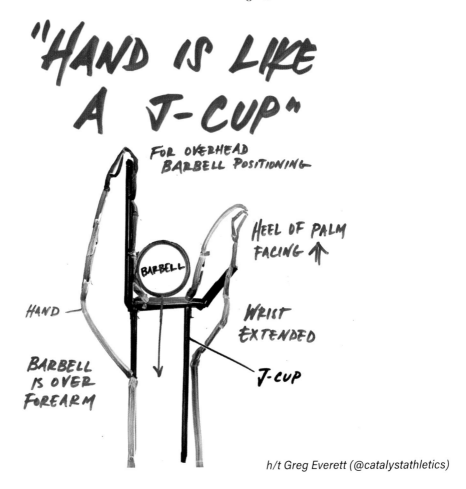

"HAND IS LIKE A J-CUP"

FOR OVERHEAD BARBELL POSITIONING

HEEL OF PALM FACING ↑

BARBELL

HAND

WRIST EXTENDED

BARBELL IS OVER FOREARM

J-CUP

h/t Greg Everett (@catalystathletics)

When?

This cue describes the hand and wrist position when holding the bar overhead.

What does this mean?

The position of the hand holding a barbell overhead should mimic that of a J-cup on a rack. The basic position follows these criteria:

- The barbell is over the forearm, slightly behind the midline.
- The wrist is in extension (not neutral).
- The heel of the palm is pointing toward the ceiling.

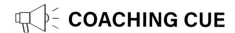
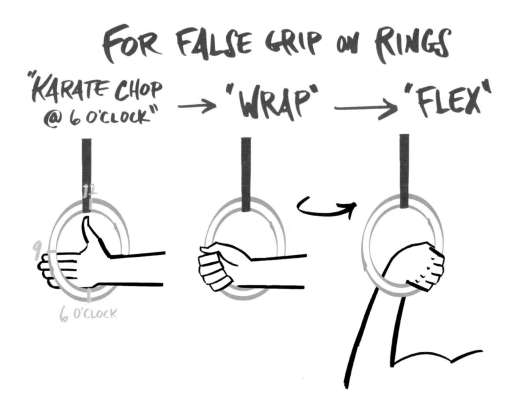

When?

This cue explains how to secure the false grip on the rings.

What does this mean?

Have the athlete "karate chop" the ring at the 6 o'clock position and then wrap their thumbs around to aggressively grip the rings as if they are flexing their forearms and biceps.

These cues teach the athlete how to keep the wrist above the ring in the hang position, which is the key to the false grip position.

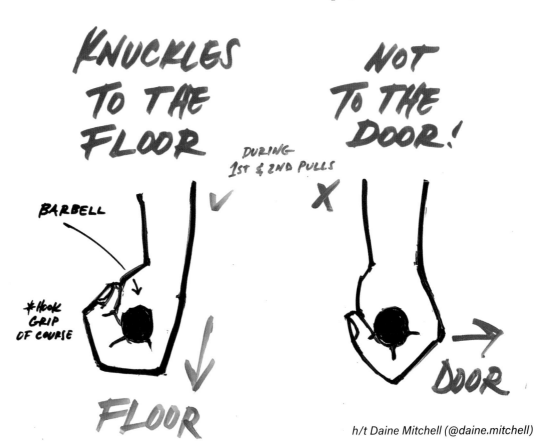

KNUCKLES TO THE FLOOR

DURING 1st & 2nd PULLS ✓

NOT TO THE DOOR! ✗

BARBELL

#HOOK GRIP OF COURSE

FLOOR ↓

DOOR →

h/t Daine Mitchell (@daine.mitchell)

When?

Use this cue to coach the first and second pulls of the clean or snatch.

What does this mean?

Pointing the knuckles down to the ground may help the athlete keep their arms extended through the first and second pulls and keep the bar close to the body.

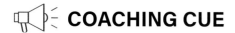 **COACHING CUE**

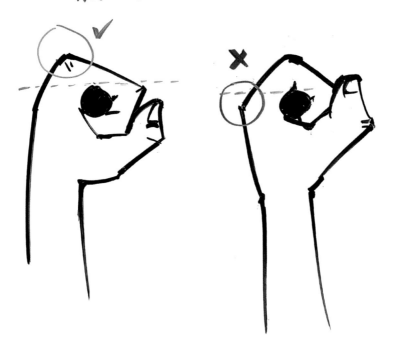

"KNUCKLES ON TOP"

WHEN GRIPPING THE PULL-UP BAR

When?
This cue describes the grip on the pull-up bar.

What does this mean?
Gripping the pull-up bar with the knuckles on top and the thumb wrapped under and around provides an optimal position for pull-ups.

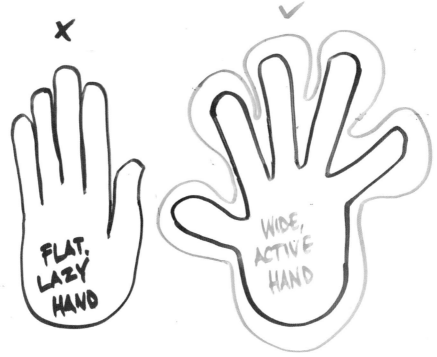

"MAKE GECKO HANDS"

x ✓

FLAT, LAZY HAND

WIDE, ACTIVE HAND

h/t Chuck Bennington (@chuckbennington)

When?

Use this cue to coach movements that involve pressing from the floor (variations of push-ups, handstand push-ups, handstand walking, etc.).

Why?

A wide active hand

- Recruits more muscles from the arm
- Is more stable
- Grabs more of the floor

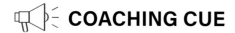
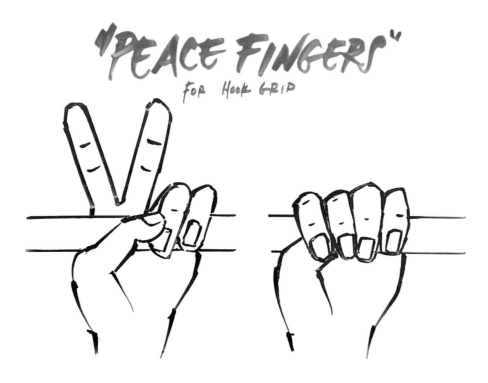

When?

Use this cue to explain the hook grip for the snatch or clean.

Why?

The hook grip is an eventual necessity to maintain control of the barbell, especially during the explosive force put on the bar during the second pull.

To establish the hook grip, the athlete presses the webbing of the hand into the bar, wraps the thumb around the bar as far as possible, and uses the first two fingers to pull the thumb farther around the bar. This grip is locked into place throughout the first and second pulls of the snatch or clean.

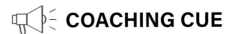
"PULL THE BAR APART"
DURING BENCH PRESS

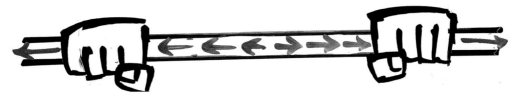

h/t Jake Boly (@jake_boly)

When?

Offer this cue while athletes are working on the bench press.

Why?

Prior to unracking the bar, the athlete tucks their shoulder blades under their back and presses their chest to the sky. When they unrack the bar, they pull their lats together. Remind them to think about pulling the bar apart and pulling their chest up to the bar as they bring the bar down.

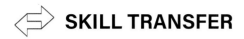

SKILL TRANSFER

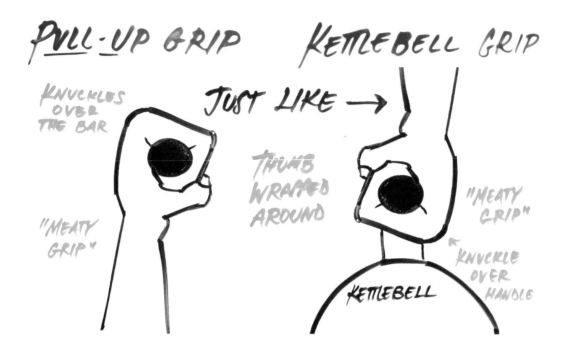

When?

Use this simple cue for teaching an effective pull-up grip by comparing it to a kettlebell grip.

Points of performance

- Knuckles are over the bar/handle.
- The thumb is wrapped around.
- The bar is held with a "meaty grip"—in the meaty part of the hand, not the fingers.

Need more help?

Watch "Gymnastics Course: Pull-Up Grip" featuring Pamela Gagnon (@pamelagnon) at https://journal.crossfit.com/article/gymnastics-course-pull-up-grip.

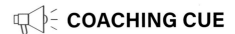

"REGRIP AT THE TOP"

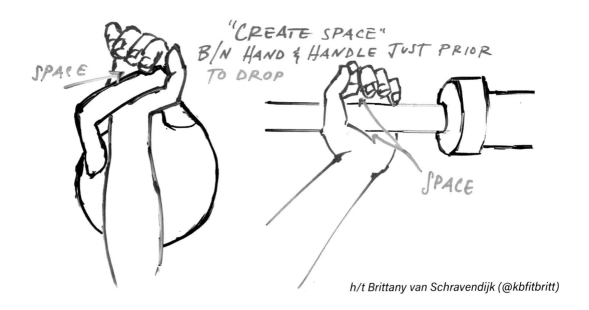

"CREATE SPACE" B/N HAND & HANDLE JUST PRIOR TO DROP

SPACE

SPACE

h/t Brittany van Schravendijk (@kbfitbritt)

When?

This cue applies when cycling kettlebell and barbell movements overhead.

What does this mean?

When cycling kettlebell and barbell movements overhead, the regrip begins at the top when the athlete creates a small space between the hand and the steel. Prior to initiating the drop back down, the kettlebell or barbell is weightless for a split second. At this moment, the athlete regrips the bar or handle and prepares for the next repetition.

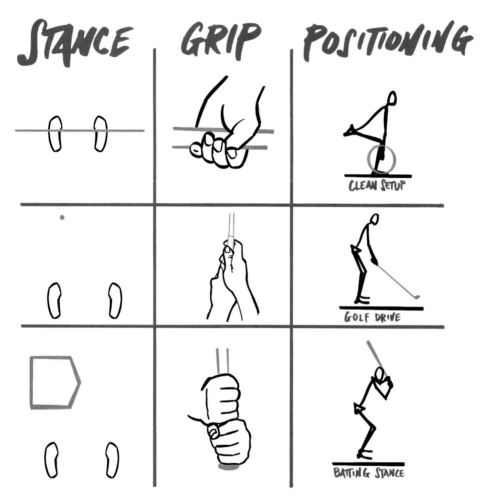

h/t Burgener Strength (@burgenerstrength)

When?

As you introduce a new movement, referencing commonalities with other familiar movements may help the athletes transfer the skills necessary to be successful.

What does this mean?

Just like other sports that involve some sort of apparatus (golf club, baseball bat, kettlebell, etc.), the fundamentals of Olympic weightlifting and the keys to successful lifts are found in the stance, grip, and positioning.

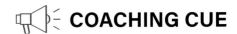
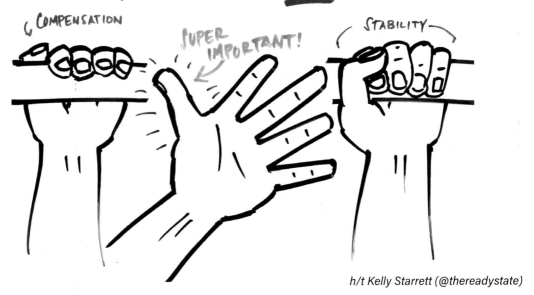

h/t Kelly Starrett (@thereadystate)

When?

This cue applies to gripping anything and everything.

What does this mean?

Wrapping the thumb creates a more stable, externally rotated position, which leads to a better connection between the arm and the body.

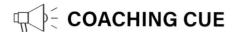
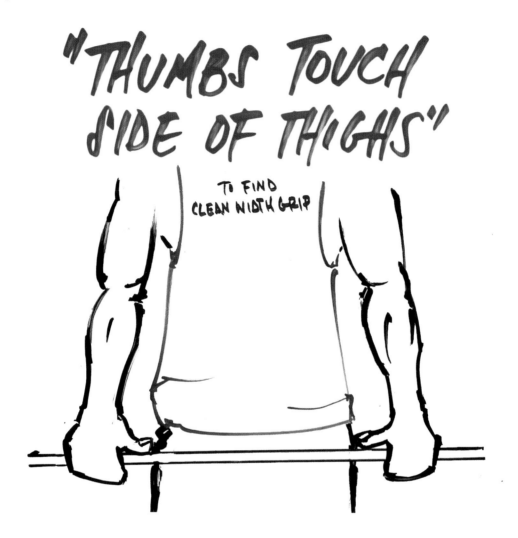

"THUMBS TOUCH SIDE OF THIGHS"

TO FIND CLEAN WIDTH GRIP

When?

This cue helps athletes find the right width of the clean grip on the barbell.

What does this mean?

The athlete should stand while holding the bar and extend their thumbs. The tips of the thumbs should touch the sides of the thighs.

CHAPTER (11)

POSITIONING

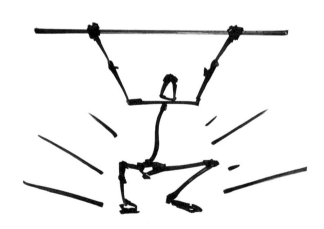

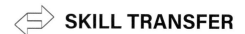
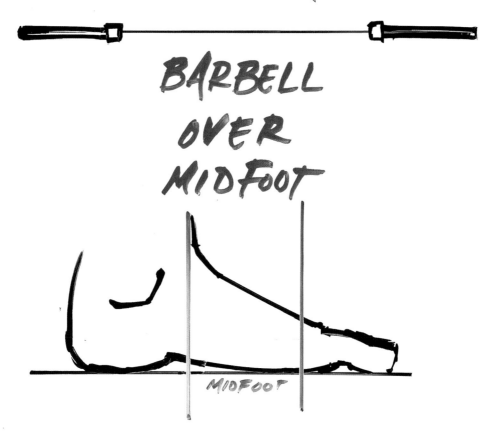

When?

This skill transfer helps athletes identify similarities among different movements and better understand body awareness.

What does this mean?

In all of the following movements, the bar should stay over the midfoot region:

- Deadlift
- Sumo deadlift
- Back squat
- Front squat
- Overhead squat
- Snatch

- Hang snatch
- Block snatch
- Power snatch
- Clean
- Hang clean
- Block clean

- Power clean
- Press
- Push press
- Push jerk
- Thruster

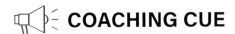

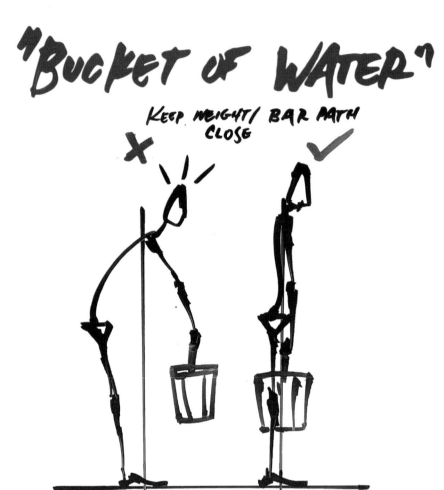

When?

This cue explains the importance of keeping the bar path close—for example, during the deadlift.

What does this mean?

A person doesn't pick up and carry a bucket of water with it far away from their body. Keeping the weight close to the body is a more efficient use of power.

Why?

Identifying similarities between everyday situations and movements in a fitness setting may help athletes gain a better sense of body awareness.

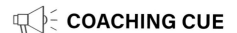
"OWN YOUR POSITION"

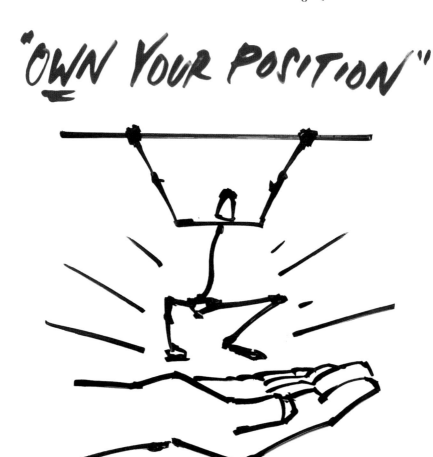

When?

This cue applies to movement of any kind.

What does this mean?

Owning your position means being able to pause and display control.

Why?

Working on "owning your position" has the following benefits:

- Builds body and spatial awareness
- Builds body control
- Builds self-confidence
- Helps identify weaknesses

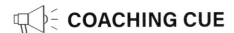
COACHING CUE

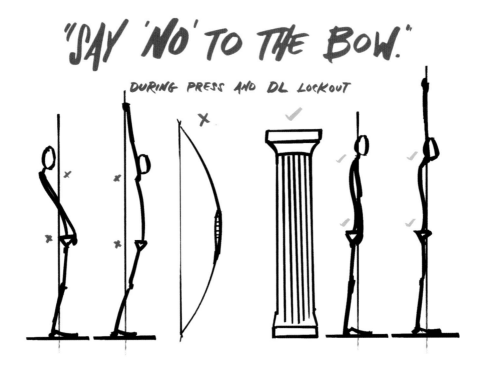

When?

This cue applies to the lockout position for the press and deadlift.

What does this mean?

Hyperextension of the back during the lockout of the press and deadlift creates a less safe, weaker position. Cue the athlete to create a strong column of support by keeping the shoulders and hips in line.

"MUTED HIP"

MOVEMENT FAULT: MUTED HIP FUNCTION

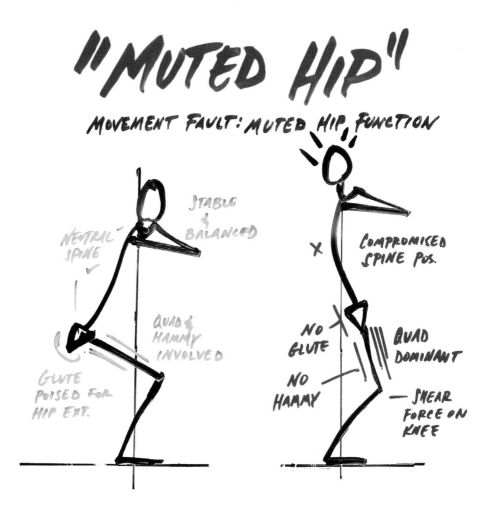

NEUTRAL SPINE ✓

STABLE & BALANCED

QUAD & HAMMY INVOLVED

GLUTE POISED FOR HIP EXT.

COMPROMISED SPINE POS.

NO GLUTE

NO HAMMY

QUAD DOMINANT

— SHEAR FORCE ON KNEE

When?

This fault occurs in many areas but most commonly during the clean receive.

What does this mean?

Muted hip results from the legs compensating for the hip's failure to flex. The most prominent effects are decreased stability, balance, and power.

CHAPTER (12)

APPROACH

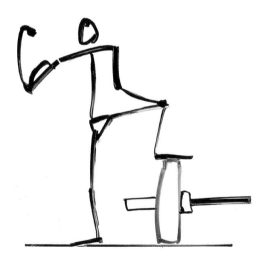

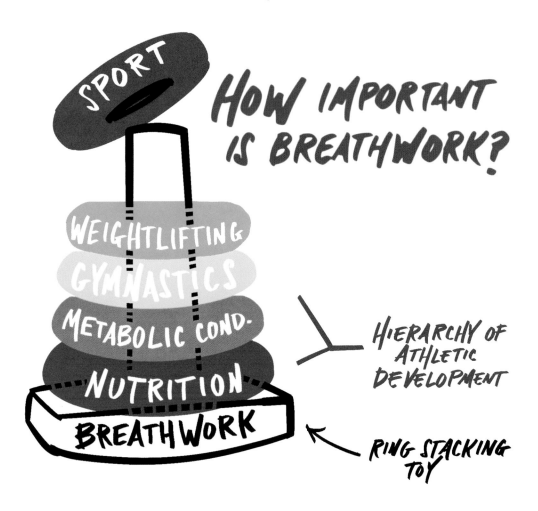

What does this mean?

Breathwork is not only the basis for the hierarchy of athletic development but also the pillar that runs through the rest of the layers, similar to the base of a toddler's ring-stacking toy. The breath affects everything from emotions to physiological and psychological performance.

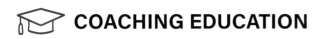
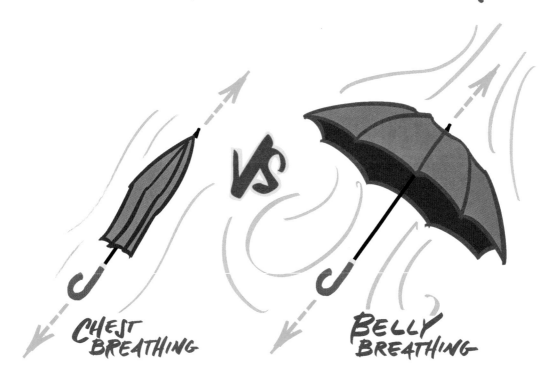

What does this mean?

A closed umbrella can't move air like an open umbrella. An athlete needs to use their diaphragm like an umbrella and open it up.

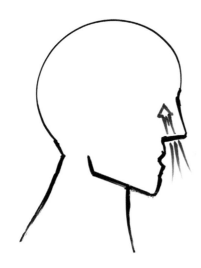

"THE NOSE KNOWS"
5 REASONS FOR NASAL BREATHING

1. PARTICLE FILTER
2. SLOWS RESPIRATION RATE DOWN
3. IMMUNE SYSTEM FIRST DEFENSE OF ALL AIR
4. HUMIDIFICATION OF AIR
5. GREATER DIAPHRAGMATIC CONTROL/USE = BETTER MECHANICAL ADVANTAGE

h/t Brian Mackenzie (@_brianmackenzie)

What does this mean?

1. The hairs and mucus in the nose act as particle filters.

2. Breathing through the nose slows down the respiration rate.

3. The immune system is the first defense of all air.

4. Breathing through the nose humidifies the air.

5. Nasal breathing provides greater diaphragmatic control and use, which gives athletes a better mechanical advantage.

"I just do it (nasal breathing) because it works."

—**SAM DANCER** (@samdancing)

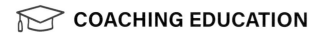

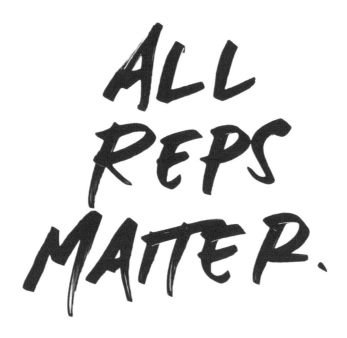

What does this mean?

Whether you realize it or not, you are training a movement pattern *every time* you move a barbell:

- Warm-up reps
- Working set reps
- Max out reps
- Competition reps

- Demonstration reps (coaches)
- "CrossFit MetCon" reps
- "Crappy" reps
- "Perfect" reps

If you want to improve your technique, don't let these opportunities pass you by.

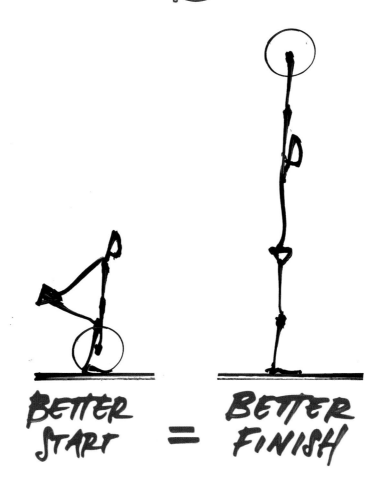

What does this mean?

A better warm-up leads to a better workout. A better setup leads to a better rep. A better plan leads to a better outcome.

Take the time to give your start the value it deserves.

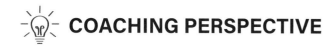

"CHEAT CODE"

⬆️⬆️⬇️⬇️⬅️➡️⬅️➡️ Ⓑ Ⓐ

CONTRA (1987)
+30 LIVES
NINTENDO ENTERTAINMENT SYSTEM

DEEP BREATH	PLACE LEFT FOOT UNDER BAR	PLACE RIGHT FOOT UNDER BAR	PLACE LEFT HAND ON BAR	PLACE RIGHT HAND ON BAR

RITUAL FOR ADDRESSING THE BAR

What does this mean?

If you're a child of the '80s and played Contra on the NES, this cheat code was a ritual. It gave you thirty lives and set you up to be as successful as possible in the game. When addressing the bar before any lift, using a ritual sets you up for success.

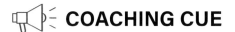

"COPY MACHINE"

MAKE YOUR LAST LIFT LOOK LIKE YOUR FIRST

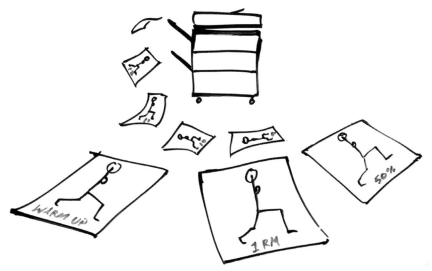

*h/t Glenn Pendlay (@glenn_pendlay) from
"Consistency in Olympic Lifting" on the On Target
Publications website*

When?

Use this cue to help athletes achieve consistency in Olympic lifting (or any movement, for that matter).

What does this mean?

Consistency with technique is one of the most important aspects of Olympic weightlifting. Athletes should try to make the last reps with heavier weight look like copies of their first reps with lighter weight.

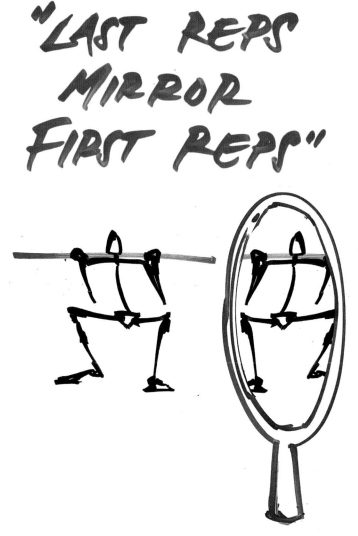

h/t Mike Dewar (@mikejdewar)

What does this mean?

The first reps of a workout are the lightest ones. The body is primed, the movements are sharp, and the technique is spot on. Throughout the workout, the body may get tired, the movements may get slow, and the technique may get sloppy. The goal should be to develop the discipline to have the last reps of the workout mirror the first reps of the workout. This will be a catalyst for improvement.

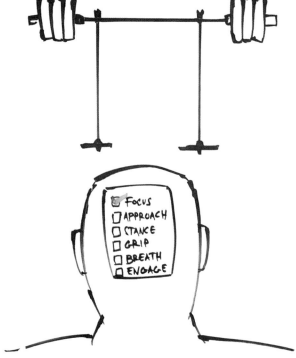

"DON'T RUSH YOUR SETUP."

h/t Westside Barbell (@westsidebarbellofficial)

When?

Use this cue to help athletes prepare for a big lift or move.

What does this mean?

Athletes should take their time with their lifts and treat each attempt as if it is the last opportunity to lift. Attention to detail in the setup will pay off during the lift.

Why?

Taking time with the setup provides

- Physical preparation
- Mental preparation
- Safety
- A routine

💡 COACHING PERSPECTIVE

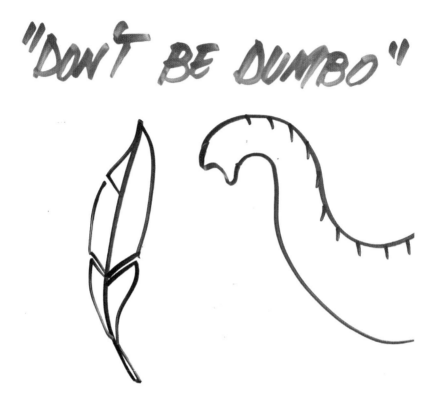

What does this mean?

Remember Dumbo, the sweet little elephant with the big ears who was convinced that he needed his magic feather to fly? Turns out he didn't need it after all.

Accessories like the following can be fantastic additions to training:

- Gymnastics grips
- Knee sleeves
- Oly shoes
- Wrist wraps
- Weight belt
- Personalized jump rope
- Lucky charm

However, don't become reliant on them. When training for general physical preparedness, the focus is likely on functional movement for real-world application. Gymnastics grips aren't always available when it's time to play with a kid on the monkey bars.

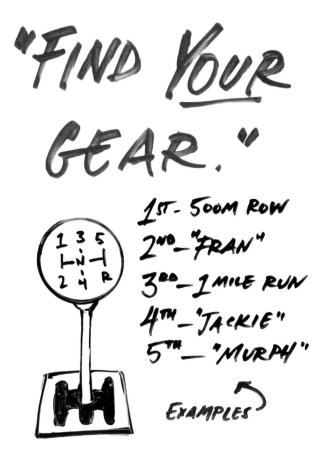

"FIND YOUR GEAR."

1ST - 500M ROW
2ND - "FRAN"
3RD - 1 MILE RUN
4TH - "JACKIE"
5TH - "MURPH"

EXAMPLES

When?

Use this cue to help athletes understand and maximize their bodies' capability during a workout.

What does this mean?

The level of an athlete's understanding of their "gears" is a direct correlation to body awareness gained from their depth of experience.

Most novice athletes have no idea what their physical abilities are and how to pace themselves. During a workout, it is important to find the right balance of work and rest so you can get the most work done before the clock runs out.

Need more help?

For more information, please read "The Thin Red Line of Fitness" by Emily Beers (coach at @madlabschooloffitness) at http://journal.crossfit.com/2014/02/the-thin-red-line-of-fitness.tpl.

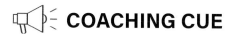 **COACHING CUE**

"LET THE WEIGHT SETTLE."

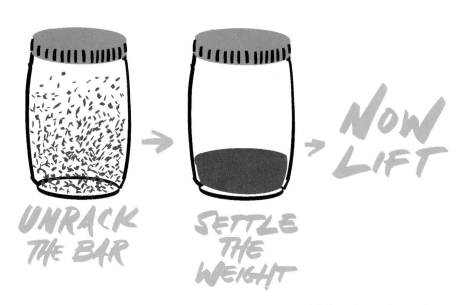

UNRACK THE BAR → SETTLE THE WEIGHT → NOW LIFT

h/t Sam Brown (@sambrownstrength)

When?

This cue applies to both squatting and bench pressing.

What does this mean?

When unracking heavy weight, even the slightest movement can negatively impact an athlete's ability to get in the best position possible. The approach should be methodical every single time:

- Unrack the weight.
- Let the weight settle and stop any kind of momentum.
- Initiate the rep.

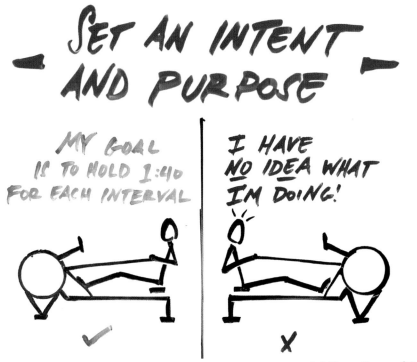

SET AN INTENT
AND PURPOSE

MY GOAL
IS TO HOLD 1:40
FOR EACH INTERVAL

I HAVE
NO IDEA WHAT
IM DOING!

h/t Shane Farmer (@shanefarmer)

What does this mean?

Prior to the workout, athletes should have a plan for what they're going to do. If they don't establish parameters, they'll likely give up earlier in the workout as things get uncomfortable. If they set a standard and expectation of themselves, they'll likely work to meet the goal.

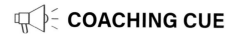 **COACHING CUE**

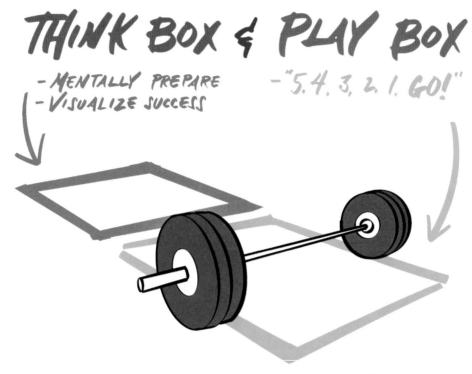

h/t Sonny Webster (@sonnywebstergb)

When?

Use this cue to help prevent overthinking during Olympic lifting.

What does this mean?

An imaginary square on the ground a few feet behind the bar can be considered the "think box." It's where the athlete does their mental preparation, thinks about technical cues, and visualizes the execution of the lift.

When the athlete is ready, they step out of the "think box" and up to the bar. They are now in the "play box," which is where they carry out what they have visualized and complete a good lift.

By setting boundaries for when to think and when to act, the athlete stays focused on what matters and when.

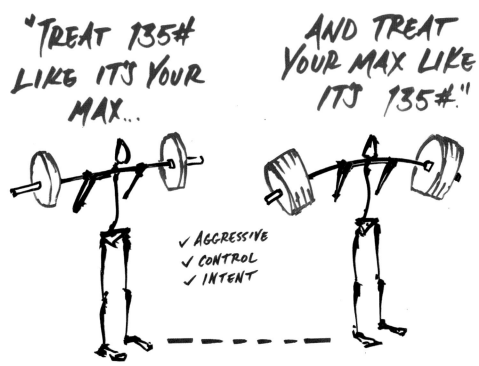

"TREAT 135# LIKE ITS YOUR MAX..."

AND TREAT YOUR MAX LIKE ITS 135#."

✓ AGGRESSIVE
✓ CONTROL
✓ INTENT

h/t Chad Wesley Smith (@chadwesleysmith) via @juggernauttraining

When?

This concept applies to all lifting.

What does this mean?

This concept is as much psychological as it is physical. Every single rep matters regardless of whether it involves a light bar during the warm-up or a one-rep max.

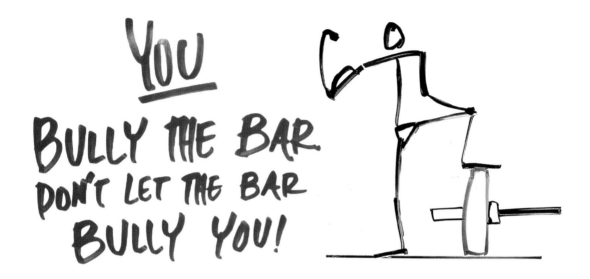

What does this mean?

During my time as a coach and an athlete, two traits that I have found to be important for success in weightlifting are aggressiveness and confidence. These traits take time to develop, but the right mentality can encourage their growth.

The perspective that I've used and shared with my athletes is to "bully the bar." I don't mean to muscle the bar without any technique but to move the bar like you own it.

YOUR LIFT STARTS HERE.

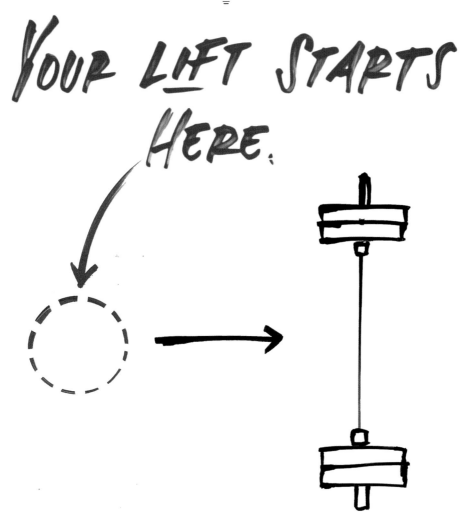

What does this mean?

A lift doesn't begin once the lifter moves the weight or even during the setup. It begins when the lifter sets their intention and walks up to the bar. The athlete must first set their mind with confidence and aggressiveness that they are going to accomplish what they set out to do. Doing so sets up the athlete for success.

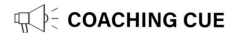
COACHING CUE

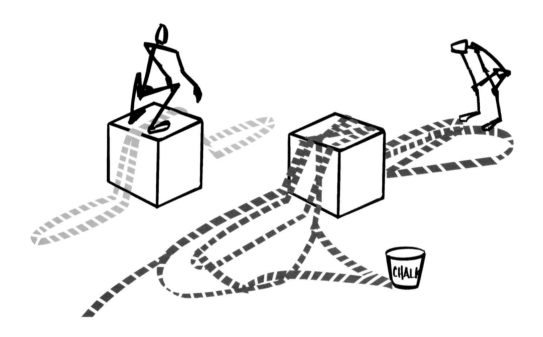

"MOVE WITH A PURPOSE."

What does this mean?

Which side of this illustration above do you fall on? If you're doing burpee box jump-overs, are you methodical and sticking to a pattern/rhythm (left)? Or do you let your feet take you wherever they want to go so that you're staggering around with no purpose (right)?

If the mind isn't focused on any sort of game plan, when fatigue hits, the athlete tends to wander around, trying to catch their breath. It wastes both time and energy. It's better to take the rest needed to stay within one's intensity threshold while staying focused and moving with a purpose.

CHAPTER (13)

PERSPECTIVES

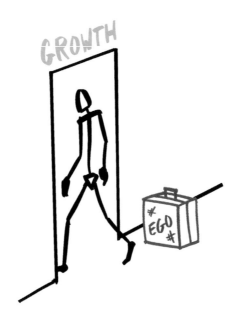

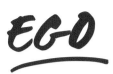

BOSS VS LEADER

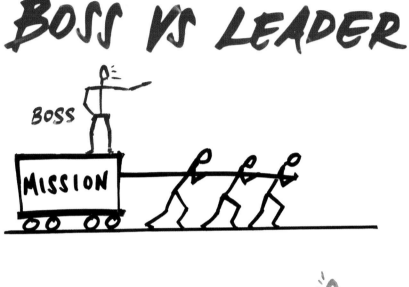

What does this mean?

A coach is tapped with the responsibility to lead athletes toward a goal, whether it is improved quality of life through nutrition and movement or optimal performance in competition.

Coaches should lead by example.

Athletes, your coach should lead by example.

This should be reflected in

- Movement standards
- Nutrition choices
- Content of character

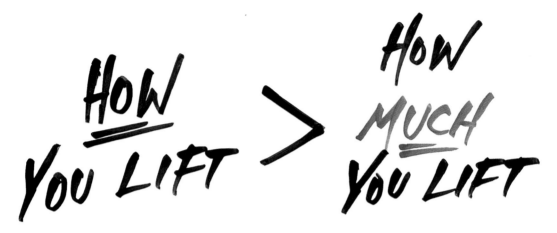

h/t Dr. Aaron Horschig (@squat_university)

What does this mean?

An athlete's goal is to lift big weights, but a more important goal is to be able to do so for the rest of one's life. *How* an athlete lifts weights is the primary factor that determines that outcome. When an athlete focuses on *how* they lift, they'll soon notice *how much more* they can lift!

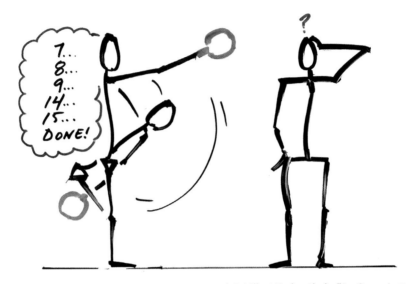

IF YOU CHEAT, YOUR COACH NOTICED.

h/t Mike Warkentin in "An Open Letter to Cheaters"

What does this mean?

Good coaches know things:

- Their athlete's ability and fitness level
- Approximately how long it takes to complete certain workouts
- How long the athlete spends working and resting

Why an athlete cheats could stem from a variety of reasons:

- They don't see cheating as a problem.
- They're lazy.
- They're embarrassed of their current fitness level.

There are no good reasons to cheat. Coaches notice, and we want you to stop.

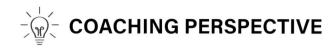

COACHING PERSPECTIVE

JUST BECAUSE YOU CAN ADD
WEIGHT / MOMENTUM
(LIFTING)   (GYMNASTICS)
DOESN'T MEAN YOU SHOULD.

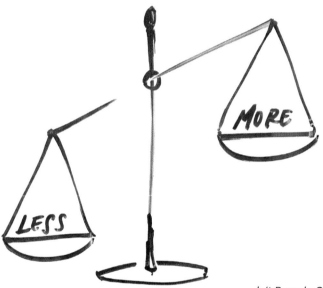

h/t Pamela Gagnon (@pamelagnon)

What does this mean?

To the beginner enthusiast, lighter weights and strict movements may not seem sexy. However, the technique gained through practicing these standards leads to proficiency and pushes the needle toward virtuosity—doing the common uncommonly well.

And virtuosity is sexy, regardless of who you are.

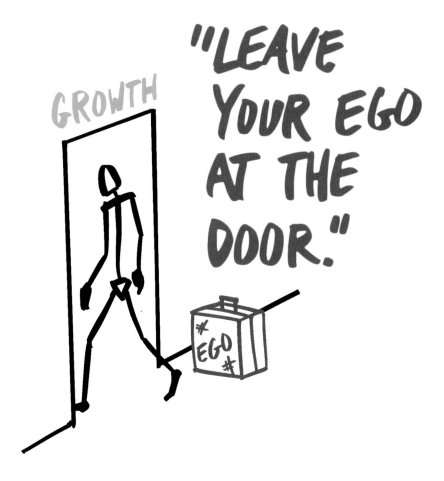

What does this mean?

The ego is a roadblock to the ability to learn, grow, and be coachable. To achieve these things, the athlete must have an open mind, a humble perspective, and a willingness to admit that they do not know everything. Leaving the ego at the door is the first step to improving.

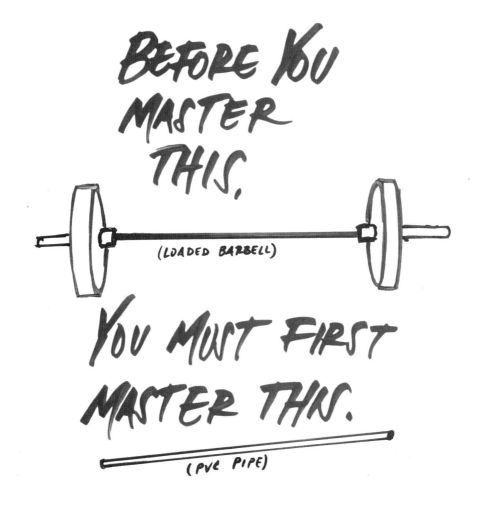

BEFORE YOU MASTER THIS,

(LOADED BARBELL)

YOU MUST FIRST MASTER THIS.

(PVC PIPE)

What does this mean?

If an athlete cannot perform a perfectly executed lift with a PVC pipe, they won't be able to do so with a loaded barbell. Proper mechanics must first be achieved. Only once they are consistently demonstrated may intensity (a loaded barbell) be introduced.

To master anything in life, first focus on the basics because mechanics lead to consistency, which leads to intensity. Do less better, and then you can do more.

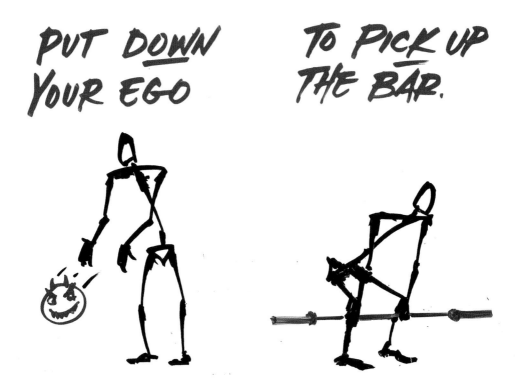

What does this mean?

I see athletes get a frustrated look when I tell them they need to take weight off the bar and focus on technique. But if a person wants to improve their lifts, they're going to have a hard time holding on to both their ego and the bar. This is likely the toughest lesson to learn, especially within Olympic weightlifting.

The truth of the matter is the more focus on technique at lighter weights (which takes patience and humility), the heavier the loads will be in the long run.

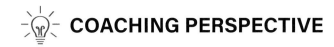
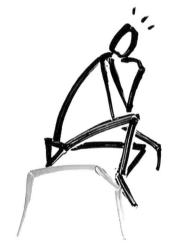

RESPONSIBILITY
RESPONSE /ABILITY

YOUR ABILITY
TO RESPOND
THE RIGHT WAY

Larry Gaier (@larry_thehuman)

What does this mean?

Coaches have a degree of accountability where their athletes are concerned. Communicating this breakdown of the word *responsibility* may help your athlete understand what it means to be responsible when it comes to training, nutrition, recovery, etc.

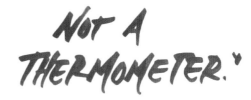
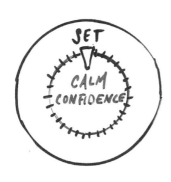

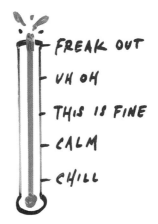

What does this mean?

A thermometer measures the temperature of the environment.

A thermostat regulates the environment.

A coach's athletes are influenced by the coach's attitude far more than by the instruction the coach gives. A coach needs to set the right environment.

Thermometer coach

- Athlete is frustrated; coach is frustrated.
- Athlete is nervous; coach is nervous.
- Athlete is disappointed; coach is disappointed.

Thermostat coach

- Athlete is frustrated; coach is calm and confident.
- Athlete is nervous; coach is calm and confident.
- Athlete is disappointed; coach is calm and confident.

WORK HARD & BE NICE TO PEOPLE.

h/t Anthony Burrill (@anthonyburrill)

What does this mean?

This simple phrase is a perspective that applies to all humans, but I think it's especially relevant to coaches:

- **Work hard:** Coaches should lead by example, constantly learning so that they can teach others. Coaches should dedicate themselves to their craft.

- **Be nice to people:** Coaches should be patient and understanding, take the time to listen and "ask a second question," and try to take on different perspectives.

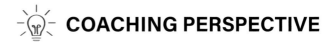
"LEADERS L.E.A.D."

LEAVE
EGO
AT THE
DOOR

h/t WUWO (@warmupandworkout)

What does this mean?

Good leaders are constantly learning from others, including those they lead. To take on this perspective, a leader must understand that they may not know everything and be willing to do what it takes to find the answer. The ego cannot exist in an open mind.

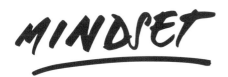
> "WHEN ANIMALS SURRENDER THEY GO LYING ON THEIR BACK.
>
> ITS A SIGN OF WEAKNESS AND SURRENDERING.
>
> I'M NEVER LYING ON MY BACK."
>
> —MIKKO SALO

What does this mean?

This quote is from the 2009 CrossFit Games champion, Mikko Salo. The Finn explained that he got this concept from an article that mentioned when animals surrender, they lie on their backs. From then on he decided he would never lie on his back after a workout because it's a sign of weakness and surrendering to the workout.

Note: To watch "Sisu—The Mikko Salo Documentary," the video where Salo says this quote, visit https://www.youtube.com/watch?v=y50JVgMEgxo.

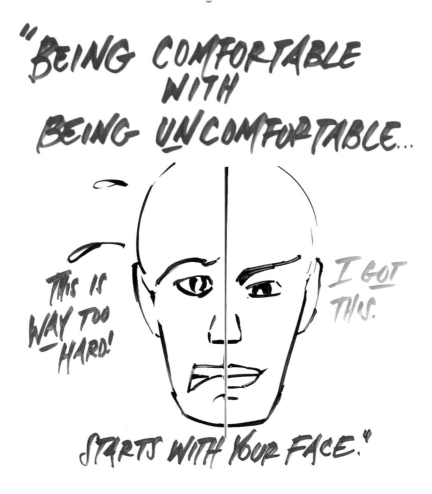

"BEING COMFORTABLE WITH BEING UNCOMFORTABLE...

THIS IS WAY TOO HARD!

I GOT THIS.

STARTS WITH YOUR FACE."

What does this mean?

The mind is a powerful tool. When an athlete makes faces of stress and defeat, they reinforce to their mind that the current challenge is indeed uncomfortable.

Athletes should work to keep a confident, determined, *comfortable* face and forget about being uncomfortable to push forward.

Don't give your mind the chance to believe that you are uncomfortable.

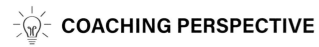
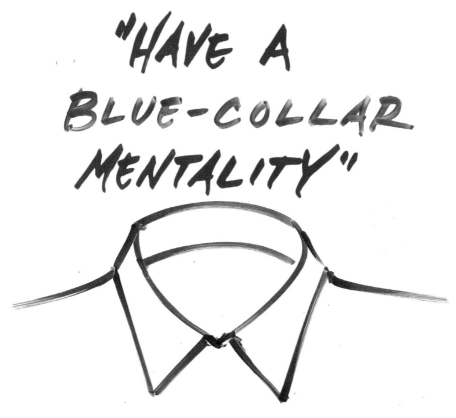

What does this mean?

Blue-collar worker refers to a person who performs physical labor and earns an hourly wage.

Applying a blue-collar mentality toward fitness means

- Clocking in every day
- Always putting forth your best effort
- Taking pride in your work
- Not being driven by the applause of others

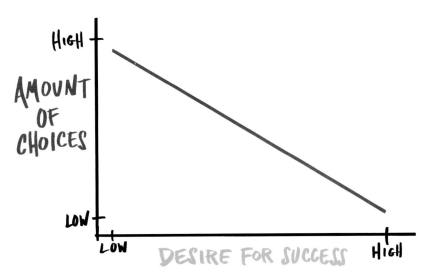
"THE HIGHER YOUR DESIRE FOR SUCCESS, THE FEWER CHOICES YOU HAVE."

h/t Zach Even-Esh (@zevenesh)

What does this mean?

Low desire for success:

- Work whenever you want.
- Rest whenever you want.
- Eat whatever you want.
- Do whatever you want.

High desire for success:

- Find a plan that's successful for you and stick with it.

"The fact of the matter is, if you want to be good, you really don't have a lot of choices because it takes what it takes.

"You have to do what you have to do to be successful. So you have to make the choices and decisions to have the discipline and focus to the process of what you need to do to accomplish your goals."

—COACH NICK SABAN

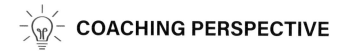

"THE HAY IS IN THE BARN."

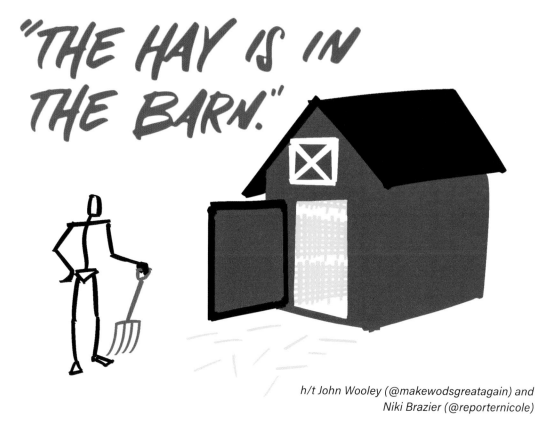

h/t John Wooley (@makewodsgreatagain) and
Niki Brazier (@reporternicole)

When?

This perspective applies to preparing for an upcoming competition.

What does this mean?

"The hay is in the barn" means all the hard work has been done. The hay has been cut, baled, and stored. There is nothing more to do.

When training for an upcoming competition, an athlete gets to the point when they've done all they can do to prepare. They may feel nervous about their performance, but they can rest assured knowing that they've done all they can do at this point. All that's left is to reap the reward of the hard work.

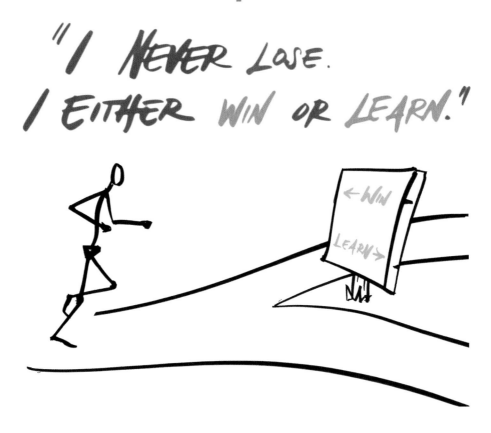

"*I NEVER LOSE.*
I EITHER WIN OR LEARN."

What does this mean?

An athlete's perspective of an impending outcome dictates how they perceive the current challenge. Understanding that they benefit either way (win or learn) helps them keep a positive mindset.

> *"I never lose. I either win or learn."*

—NELSON MANDELA

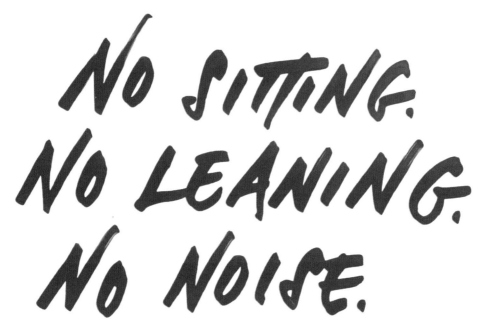

h/t Greg Everett (@catalystathletics)

When?

This perspective applies to behavior after hard conditioning.

What does this mean?

After hard conditioning, fight the urge to lean over, sit down, or even make noise. None of those actions make an athlete stronger. Furthermore, fighting the urge creates discipline and small victories that help build confidence.

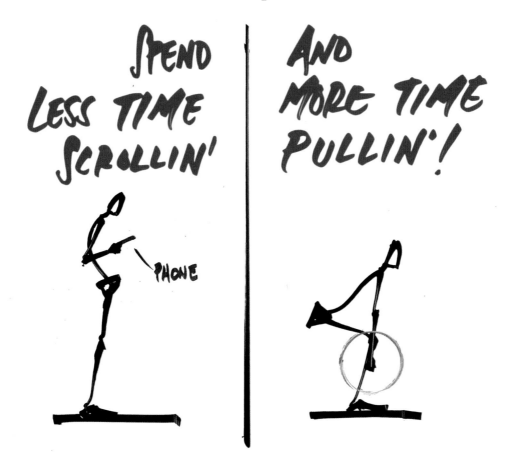

SPEND LESS TIME SCROLLIN' | *AND MORE TIME PULLIN'!*

PHONE

What does this mean?

Athletes should feel free to spend all the time they want mindlessly scrolling through a perpetual feed of distractions *outside* of the gym, but training deserves athletes' full focus. They should put down the phone, pick up the barbell (or dumbbell, kettlebell, pull-up bar, etc.), and show some *value* to gym time.

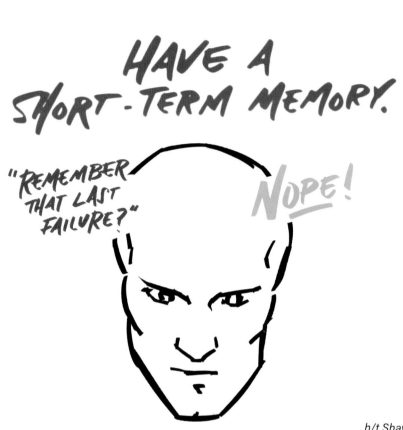

h/t Shayne McGowan
(@mental_edge_performance)

When?

Use this cue to help athletes keep confidence levels high.

What does this mean?

Learning from mistakes is good. Dwelling on them doesn't help. Having a short-term memory allows people to let go of mistakes and keep confidence at a high level. When an error occurs, acknowledge it and immediately move on.

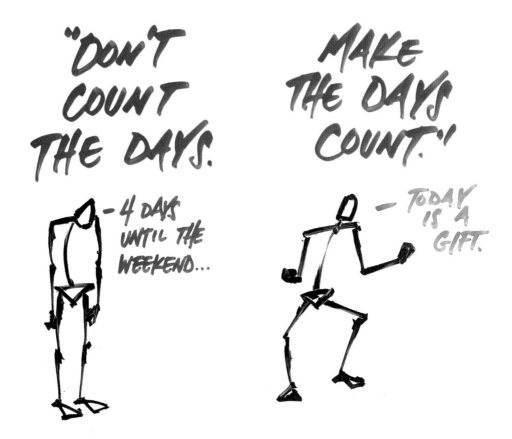

"DON'T COUNT THE DAYS."

— 4 DAYS UNTIL THE WEEKEND...

MAKE THE DAYS COUNT."

— TODAY IS A GIFT.

What does this mean?

Each day is a gift. Don't waste the days away by counting them down until the weekend. Find a passion and a purpose. Use the days to pursue those things that matter.

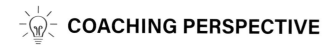
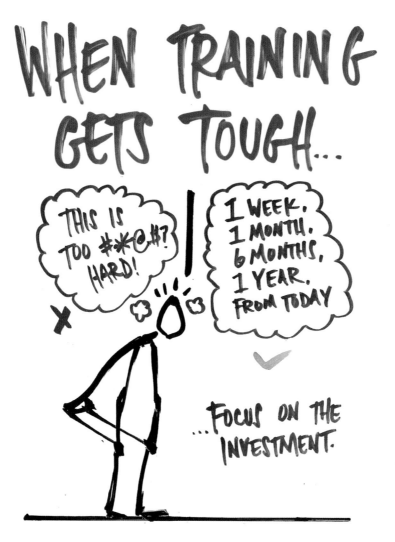

What does this mean?

When training gets tough, focus on the investment. It's easy to lose focus when

- You're out of breath (distraction).

- Your muscles are sore (distraction).

- The weight feels heavier than it is (distraction).

Instead, shift your focus to

- Why you showed up

- Where this hard work is taking you

- How you'll feel once you've accomplished your goal

WHERE IS YOUR FOCUS

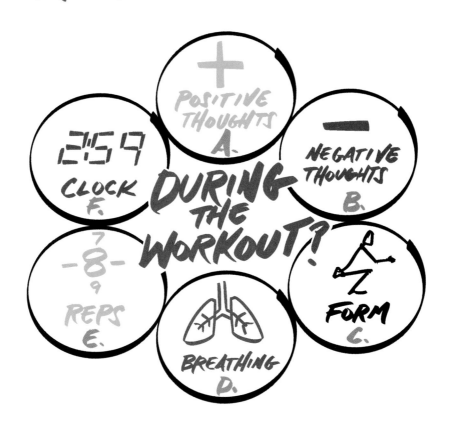

POSITIVE THOUGHTS
A.

NEGATIVE THOUGHTS
B.

FORM
C.

BREATHING
D.

REPS
E.

CLOCK
F.

DURING THE WORKOUT?

What does this mean?

Where athletes place their focus during a workout can have a major influence on the outcome of their performance. Be sure to give attention to what matters most.

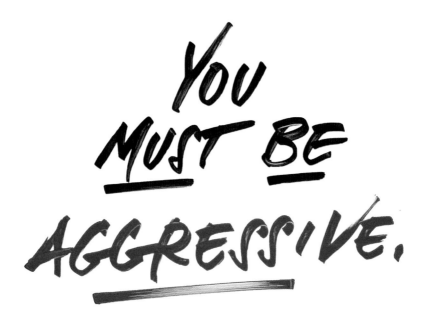

h/t Mike Dewar (@mikejdewar)

When?

This perspective is helpful when lifting heavy weight.

What does this mean?

Athletes can't just "kinda want it."

When moving heavy loads, especially during powerlifting or Olympic weightlifting, they must not only want it bad but *also* have the confidence that it *belongs* to them and they're going to take it. Anything less, and they'll get crushed.

Athletes *must* be aggressive.

MOVEMENT

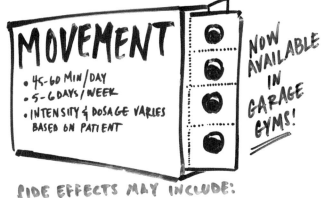

"MOVEMENT IS THE BEST MEDICINE"

ASK YOUR COACH IF MOVEMENT IS RIGHT FOR YOU.

MOVEMENT
- 45-60 MIN/DAY
- 5-6 DAYS/WEEK
- INTENSITY & DOSAGE VARIES BASED ON PATIENT

NOW AVAILABLE IN GARAGE GYMS!

SIDE EFFECTS MAY INCLUDE:
- IMPROVED QUALITY OF LIFE
- INCREASE IN MUSCLE
- DECREASE IN BODY FAT
- LOWER HR, LOWER LDL, HIGHER HDL
- FEELINGS OF CONFIDENCE AND ACCOMPLISHMENT

What does this mean?

Coaches and athletes work together to decide if movement is the right prescription:

- Suggested dosage: 45 to 60 minutes a day, 5 to 6 days a week.
- Intensity of dosage varies based on the individual.
- For best results, incorporate a diet of whole foods.
- Available at garage gyms!

Side effects may include

- Improved quality of life
- Increase in muscle, decrease in body fat
- Lower heart rate, lower LDL, increased HDL
- Feelings of confidence and accomplishment

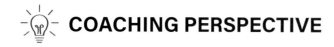

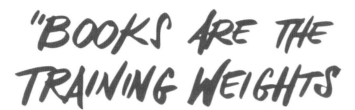

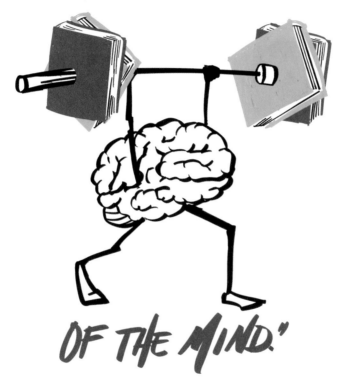

What does this mean?

The mind needs training, too. Reading books is one way to train the mind.

COACHING PERSPECTIVE

WE DON'T STOP MOVING BECAUSE WE GROW OLD.
WE GROW OLD BECAUSE WE STOP MOVING.

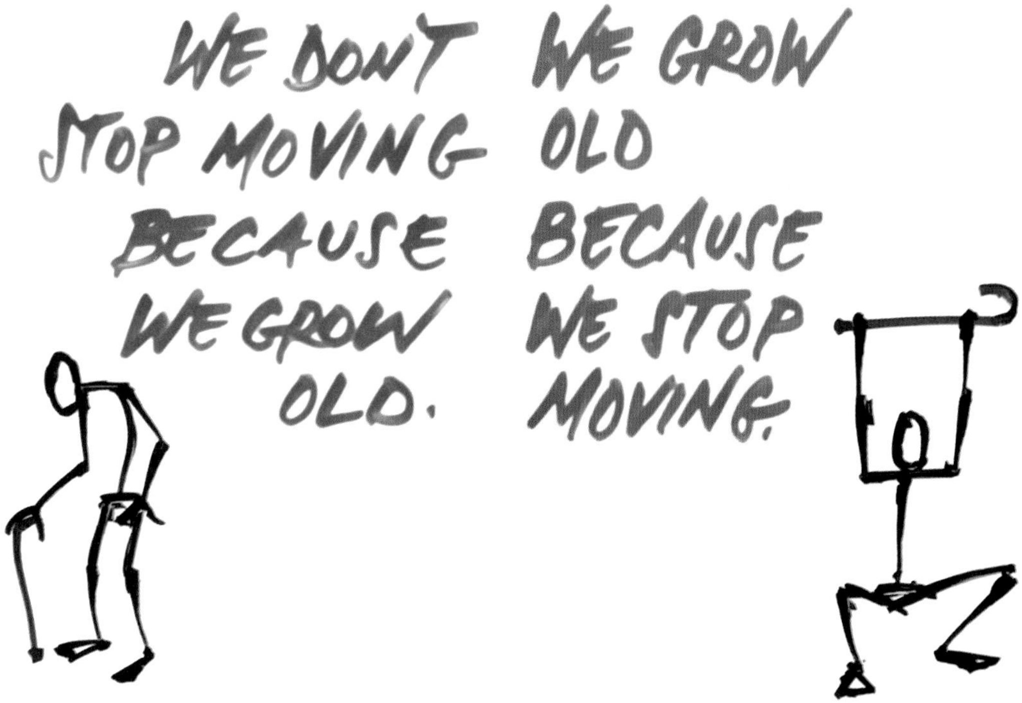

What does this mean?

You were given this beautiful body that was built to move. Use it!

> *"Every day you don't squat is one day closer to the day you can't squat."*

—**GREG EVERETT** (@catalystathletics)

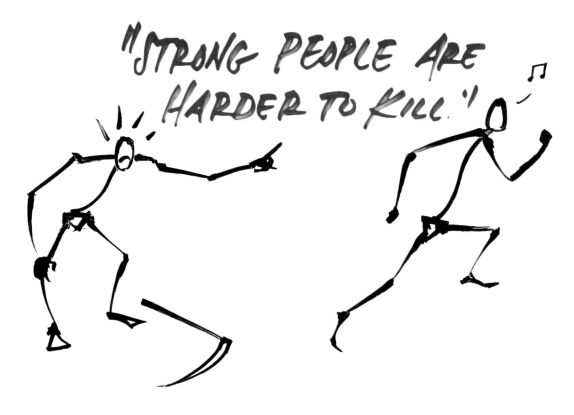

What does this mean?

Each person has only one life.
Get strong. Be useful to others.

> *"Strong people are harder to kill than weak people and more useful in general."*

—COACH MARK RIPPETOE
(@wichitafallsathleticclub)

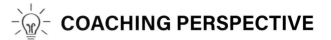
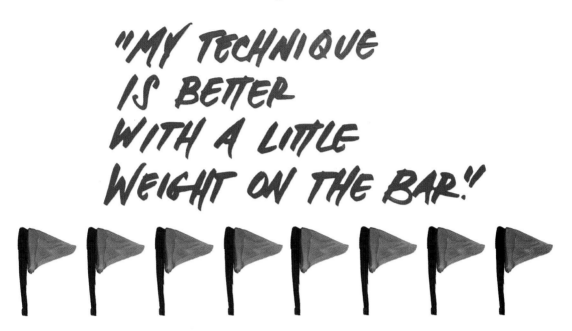

"MY TECHNIQUE IS BETTER WITH A LITTLE WEIGHT ON THE BAR."

What does this mean?

Athletes with this perspective are likely masking a technique and mobility issue that is keeping them from improving. Working with a PVC pipe provides a massive benefit because the athlete can spend time in proper positions, especially the areas where they are weak and uncomfortable, without having to worry about weight.

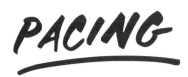 PACING

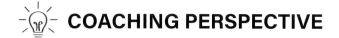 💡 **COACHING PERSPECTIVE**

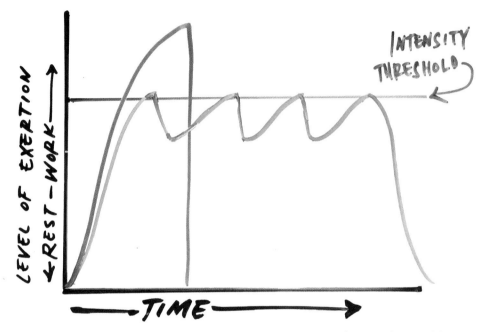

h/t Pat Sherwood (@sherwood215)

What does this mean?

Simply put, when athletes learn to manage their personal tolerance of work-to-rest ratio, they set themselves up for success.

"BREAK THE BAND"

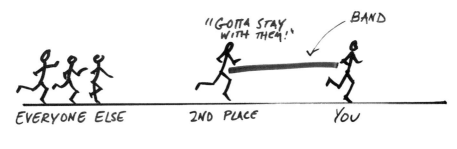

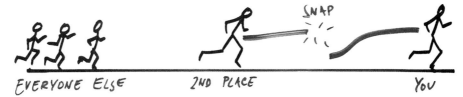

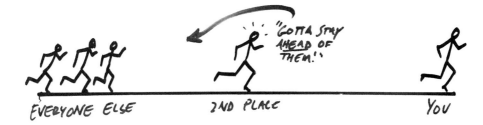

h/t Jason Khalipa (@jasonkhalipa)

What does this mean?

This perspective is based on the theory that during competition, there is an imaginary band that the competitor behind you has lassoed around you. Their focus is on you—keeping up with and catching you. The idea is to break the band and move yourself so far ahead of them that they forget about keeping up with and catching you. Instead, they shift their focus on staying ahead of the competition behind them.

This mentality can apply to business as well as sporting competition.

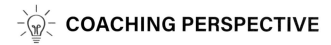

COACHING PERSPECTIVE

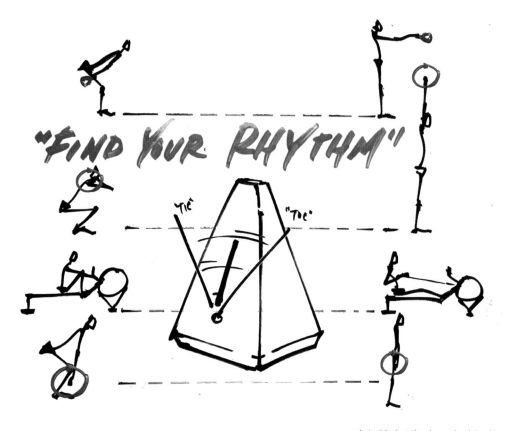

h/t Chris Hinshaw (@hinshaw363)

What does this mean?

An athlete should match the cadence of their movement to complement a consistent breathing pattern.

Why?

The body operates best when a consistent and efficient breathing pattern is established. If movement is erratic, breathing will soon become erratic, too. Find and implement the optimal movement rhythm to complement a consistent breathing pattern.

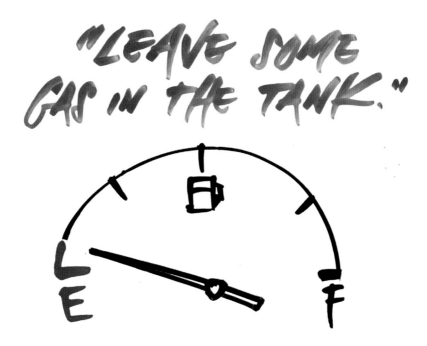

h/t Eric John (@ericejw163) at @nypd_crossfit

What does this mean?

During a training session, it's important to push yourself. However, it's more important to be able to come back the next day. Going high intensity day after day will soon lead to overtraining, plateaus in progress, and eventually injury. Know when to push yourself, but also learn when to leave a little gas in the tank.

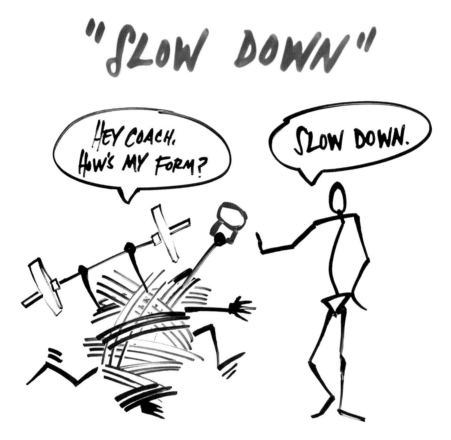

h/t Eric Cressey (@ericcressey)

What does this mean?

To become a better mover, simply slow down to become smooth and balanced. Moving is a skill that takes time, practice, and patience. Just like slowing down when you're reading or driving a car, slowing down as you move will allow your mind and body the opportunity to create good habits.

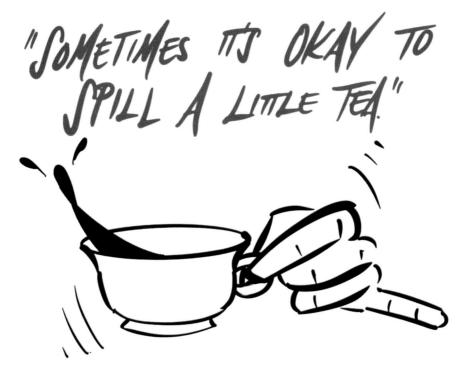
"Sometimes it's okay to spill a little tea."

h/t Jason Ackerman (@coachjasonackerman)

What does this mean?

During a Whiteboard Weekly podcast, Jason Ackerman and I were discussing the drawing "Move with a Purpose" (page 280) and how it relates not only to specific movement patterns but also to technique versus intensity. We talked about three athletes:

- The athlete who moves so perfectly that angels shed a tear.

- The athlete who is so out of control they are going to injure themselves or someone else in the class.

- The athlete who has some minor movement flaws but will be able to improve those faults with effective coaching.

That's the idea behind "sometimes it's okay to spill a little tea." An athlete who makes mistakes but can improve them has the appropriate balance of technique versus intensity. It's NOT technique OR intensity; an athlete needs both to improve their fitness. If they're not "spilling a little tea" once in a while, they aren't pushing the boundaries of their fitness level.

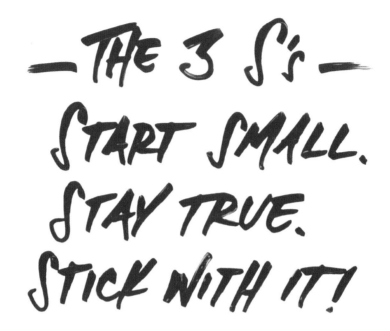

THE 3 S's —
START SMALL.
STAY TRUE.
STICK WITH IT!

When?

This perspective applies to working one's way through a project or toward a goal (fitness, business, personal, anything…).

What does this mean?

Start small. You have everything you need to get started *right now.*

Stay true. Remember why you started and stay focused.

Stick with it. Consistency is king.

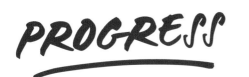 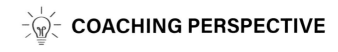

PROGRESS   COACHING PERSPECTIVE

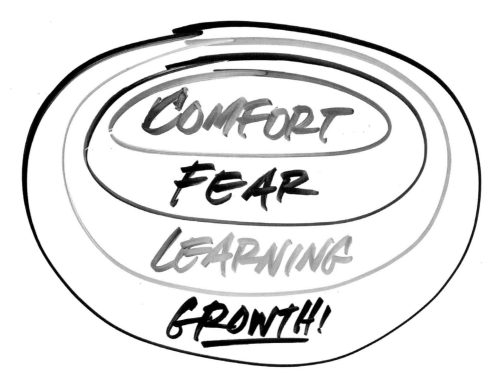

What does this mean?

Although this graphic will not correspond to every situation for everyone, there is a lot of truth in this process.

Comfort zone: Feeling safe, unchallenged, in control
Fear zone: Feeling uncertainty, lacking confidence, making excuses
Learning zone: Acquiring new skills to deal with challenges
Growth zone: Achieving and setting new goals, developing confidence

Why?

It is necessary to gain the understanding that many times fear is part of the process of growth.

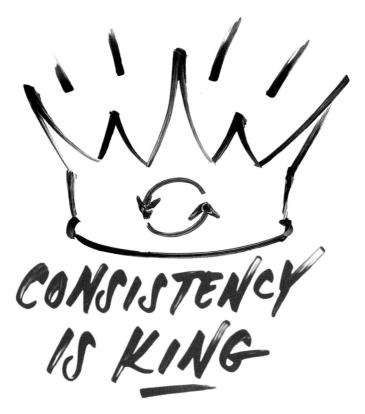

h/t Chad Vaughn (@olychad)

What does this mean?

Practicing 10 perfect reps 5 days a week is far more beneficial than pushing through 50 reps 1 day a week. The small percentage of improvement that you experience during each training session builds up over time to result in large gains. Consistency builds habits. Habits create a lifestyle. Your lifestyle determines your success.

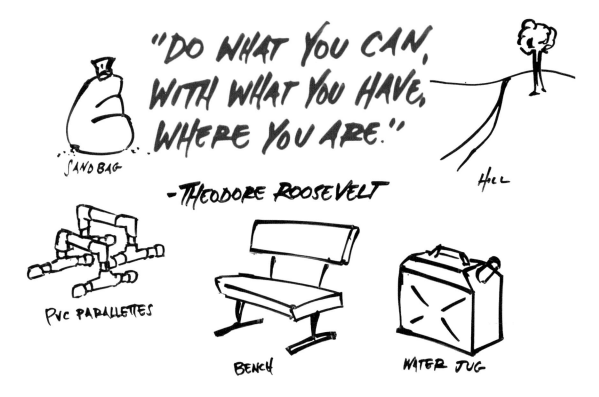

What does this mean?

You don't need expensive equipment or a fancy gym to get in shape. Some of the best athletes throughout history have accomplished far more than you with far fewer opportunities. If you want it bad enough, you'll find a way. It all comes down to discipline.

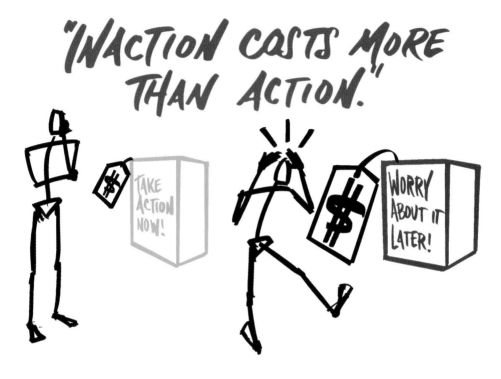

h/t Larry Gaier (@larry_thehuman)

What does this mean?

The long-term cost of not doing anything to remedy a situation is greater than what it would cost to take immediate action. This concept proves to be true in many situations, including environmental issues, business development, and especially chronic disease.

MICRO GOALS LEAD TO MAJOR GOALS!

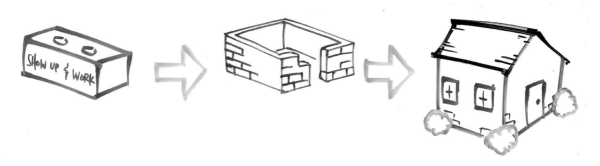

h/t Derby City CrossFit (@derbycitycf)

What does this mean?

Tiny efforts over time can lead to the accomplishment of major goals, just as a house is built brick by brick. Set appropriate micro goals that will lead to a major goal. Celebrate micro successes along the way to keep moving forward!

COACHING PERSPECTIVE

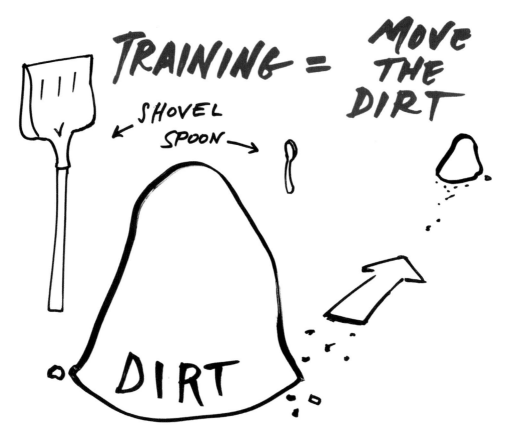

h/t John Welbourn (@johnwelbourn)

When?

This perspective may help athletes understand the importance of consistency and dedication.

What does this mean?

In simple terms, training is like moving a large pile of dirt. You will have good days when you make some serious progress and move the dirt with a shovel. You will also have bad days when you get frustrated or injured and move the dirt with a spoon. The important thing is, regardless of whether you have a shovel or a spoon, you show up every day and keep moving the dirt.

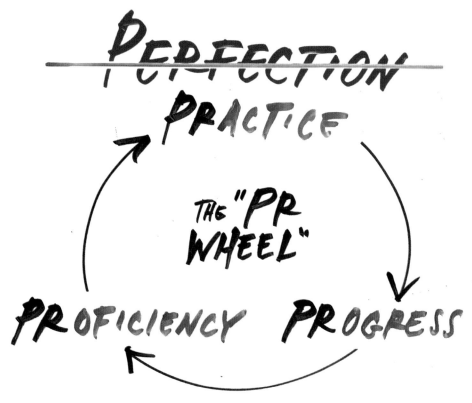

h/t Kevin Bang (@kevinbang327) of @crossfitdistinction

What does this mean?

Practice

- Pick a movement that you want to improve.
- Video yourself doing the movement.
- Ask for feedback from a coach.
- Develop a strategy to focus on technique through progressions.

Progress

- Document your progress with video, journaling, and/or frequent coaching assessment.
- Continue to practice while turning up the intensity on the movement in workouts.

Proficiency

- Compare your current state of proficiency to your past progress.
- Continue to fine-tune the elements developed through progress.

COACHING PERSPECTIVE

ATHLETE: HEY COACH,
HOW DO I GET
BETTER AT ________?

ME: PRACTICE!

What does this mean?

There is no magic pill, secret trick, or hack. Practice is the key.

Practice takes

- Effort
- Time
- Consistency
- Motivation
- Discipline
- Thoughtful movement

Leonardo da Vinci didn't get better at painting by finding some gimmicky technique on social media. Da Vinci got better at painting because he painted A LOT.

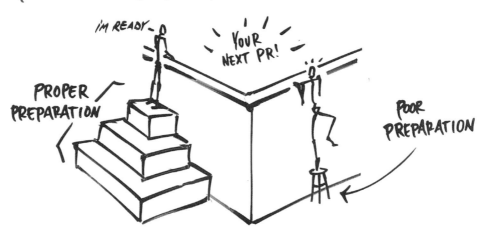

What does this mean?

Notable accomplishments rarely happen by chance. An athlete can increase the likelihood of success by taking the time and effort to create and follow a well-thought-out plan.

Remember this when it comes to

- Setting a goal
- Training for a competition
- Working toward a new PR

> "Proper preparation prevents poor performance."
>
> —MILITARY ADAGE

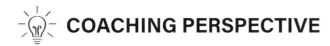
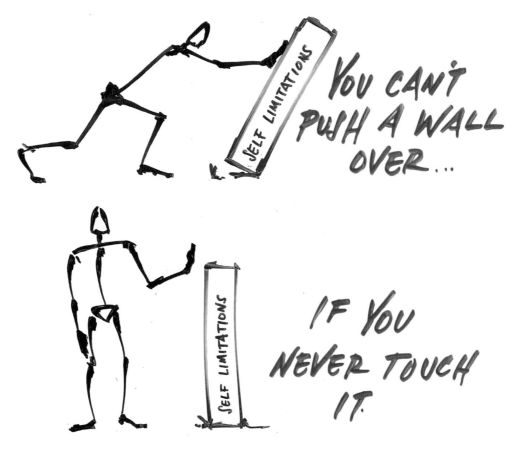

What does this mean?

The "wall" may represent many things: self limitations, previous personal bests, lofty goals, etc. Never touching the wall lets the wall win. An athlete will never gain any progress unless they

- Get familiar with the wall
- Test it
- Test themself

Then, when they're ready, the athlete can push that damn wall over!

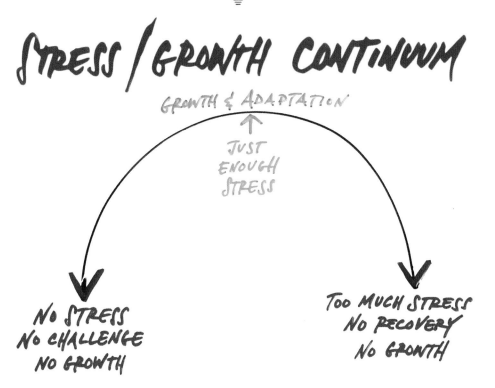

STRESS / GROWTH CONTINUUM

GROWTH & ADAPTATION

JUST ENOUGH STRESS

NO STRESS
NO CHALLENGE
NO GROWTH

TOO MUCH STRESS
NO RECOVERY
NO GROWTH

When?

Use this simple illustration to help communicate the importance of the right amount of stress (growth/recovery).

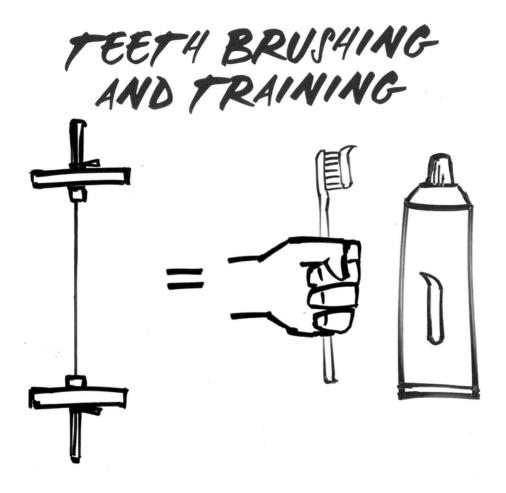

TEETH BRUSHING AND TRAINING

What does this mean?

Exercise should be a part of a person's normal routine, just like brushing their teeth is.

A person shouldn't need constant motivation to exercise. It should come naturally because it's good for the body, and it makes a person feel better after doing it.

In this illustration, the barbell represents any enjoyable healthy activity: kettlebell, hiking, running, and so on.

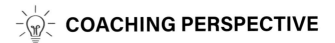
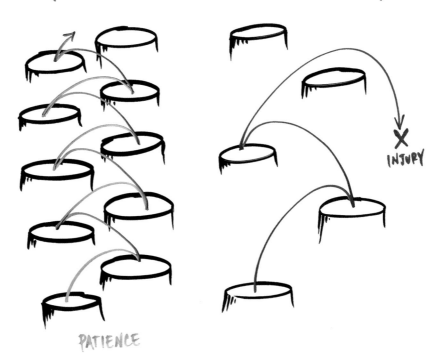

"THE SMALLER THE STEPS, THE LONGER THE JOURNEY."

h/t Larry Gaier (@larry_thehuman)

What does this mean?

Everyone wants to see progress. When you begin to see the slightest improvement, it's easy to want to make bigger jumps, thinking that it will shorten the distance to the goal. In reality, it's important to continue to make the smaller steps that will allow adaptations to stay abreast of the loads you place on yourself.

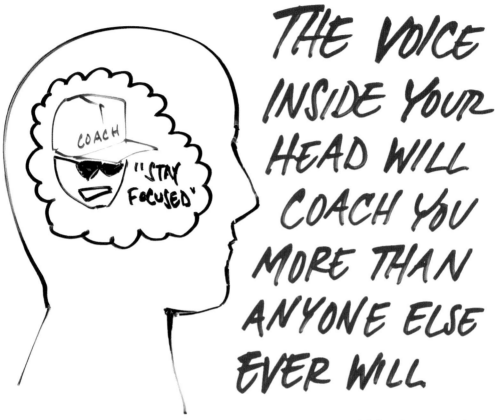

THE VOICE INSIDE YOUR HEAD WILL COACH YOU MORE THAN ANYONE ELSE EVER WILL

h/t Ben Bergeron (@benbergeron)

What does this mean?

You can have the best coaches in the world, but you'll hear no voice more than the one that is inside of your head. That voice has more influence on you than anyone else in your life. Become aware of that voice. Understand that your thoughts become your words, and your words soon become your actions. If you change the way you think, you can change the way you compete.

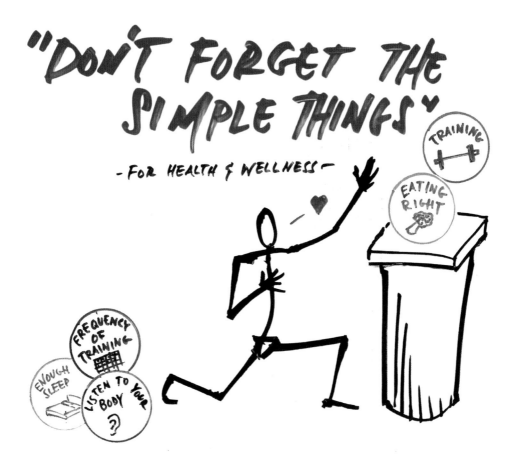

"DON'T FORGET THE SIMPLE THINGS"

— FOR HEALTH & WELLNESS —

TRAINING

EATING RIGHT

FREQUENCY OF TRAINING

ENOUGH SLEEP

LISTEN TO YOUR BODY ?

h/t Ben Bergeron (@benbergeron)

What does this mean?

Health and wellness really come down to a few simple ingredients: exercise, diet, and rest. In today's world, it's easy to get caught up in trends, life hacks, and fancy gimmicks with the hope that these things will quickly bring you closer to your goal. If you put more attention into the basics, you will soon find lasting success.

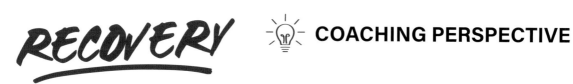

RECOVERY

COACHING PERSPECTIVE

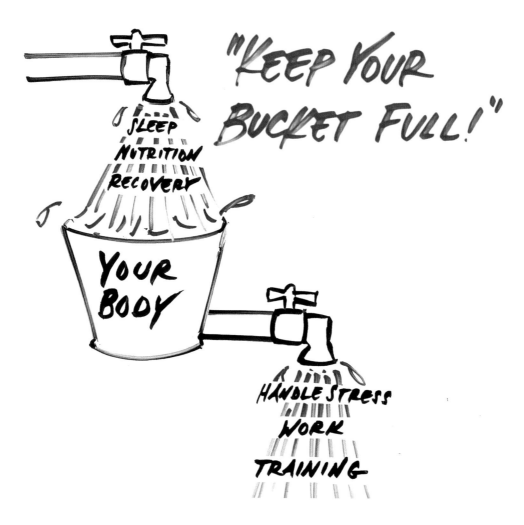

"KEEP YOUR BUCKET FULL!"

SLEEP
NUTRITION
RECOVERY

YOUR BODY

HANDLE STRESS
WORK
TRAINING

When?

This drawing helps illustrate the importance of nutrition, recovery, and sleep.

What does this mean?

A full bucket means

- Increased performance
- Increased awareness
- Increased energy
- Decreased chance of injury

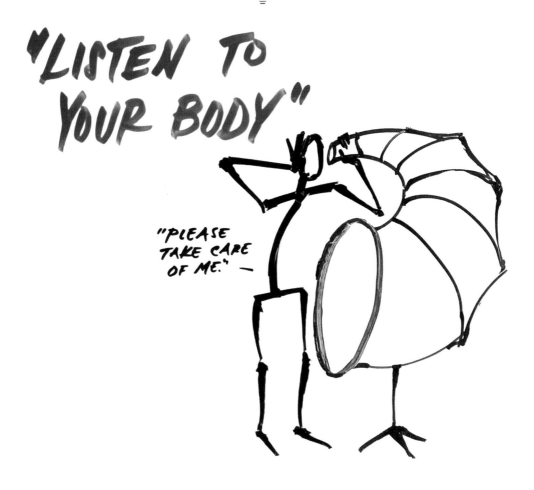

"LISTEN TO YOUR BODY"

"PLEASE TAKE CARE OF ME." —

illustration inspired by Erik Eagleman (@erikeagleman)

What does this mean?

Take a moment to slow down your movement and thoughts. Check in with yourself by asking questions:

- How am I feeling emotionally/psychologically/physically?
- What are the things that I can control?
- How are my energy levels?

As life gets busy, it's important to refocus your attention on what is important.

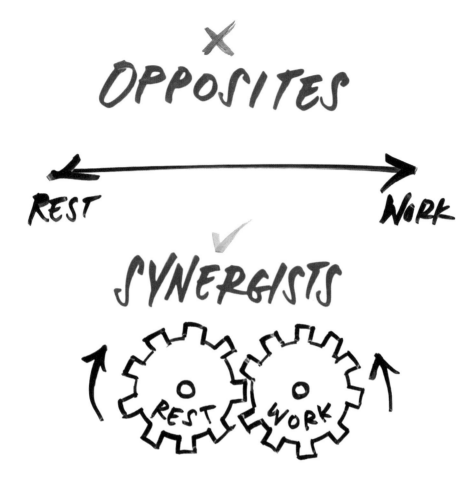

h/t Dr. Jade Teta (@jadeteta)

What does this mean?

Work and rest are not opposites. They work together as synergists. The more you rest, the harder you are able to work.

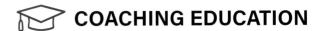

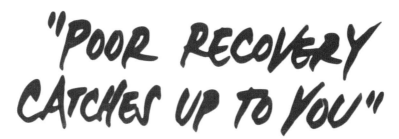

"POOR RECOVERY CATCHES UP TO YOU"

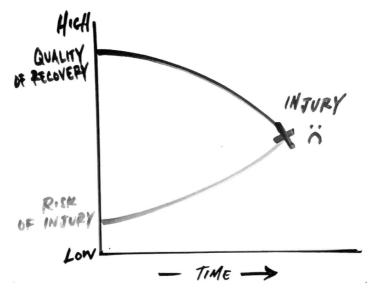

h/t Dr. Aaron Horschig (squat_university)

What does this mean?

You can get by with poor recovery for a short time, but eventually it will catch up with you and result in stagnated progress and/or injury.

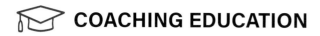
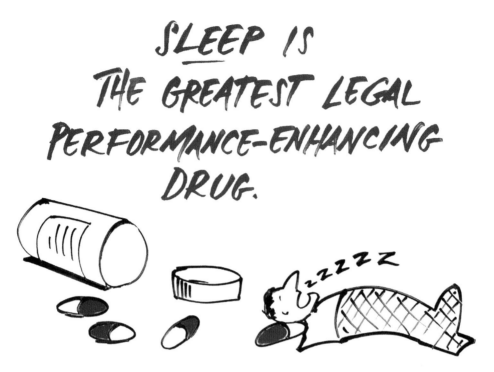

What does this mean?

Sleep is the single most important thing you can do to reset your body and brain each day. For more information, read *Why We Sleep: Unlocking the Power of Sleep and Dreams* by Matthew Walker.

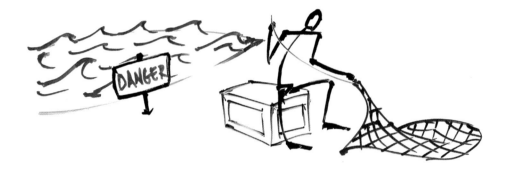

"WHEN FISHERMEN CAN'T GO TO SEA, THEY MEND THEIR NETS."

h/t Zach Long (@thebarbellphysio)

What does this mean?

Sometimes, circumstances are such that a workout routine is altered—for example, when the world shut down at the start of the COVID-19 pandemic. How an athlete gets through a time like that is up to them. Is the time a setBACK or a setUP for better things to come?

I encourage athletes to view downtime as a massive opportunity to "mend their nets." Focus on areas of fitness, especially those that may have been neglected in the past:

- Mobility
- Content knowledge
- Bodyweight movements
- Diet

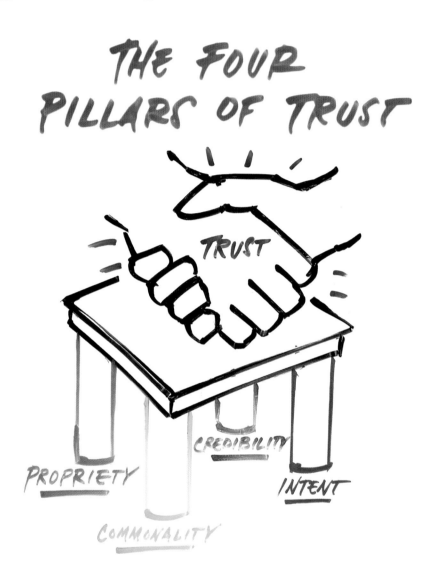

THE FOUR PILLARS OF TRUST

TRUST

PROPRIETY

COMMONALITY

CREDIBILITY

INTENT

h/t Larry Gaier (@larry_thehuman) via @activelifeprofessional

What does this mean?

If you do not establish trust with your athlete, you will never have the opportunity to exert your influence as a coach.

Trust is *earned* intentionally and deliberately. How do you build trust?

- **Propriety:** Own the part. Do you look, sound, smell, and move like the kind of professional you are?

- **Commonality:** Everyone is waiting to be seen, heard, and understood. Do you understand the other person's perspective?

- **Credibility:** Know your stuff. Understand where the other person is and where they want to be. Understand the steps to get them there.

- **Intent:** This is your "why." Everyone can smell your intent. Do you want to just make money or actually help others?

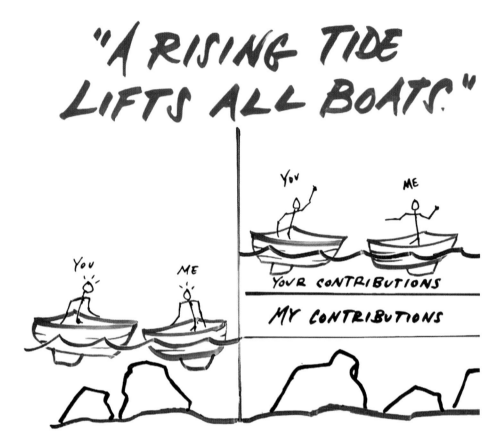

What does this mean?

This is a simple way of saying, "When I help you, and you help me, we both achieve more." This perspective may help coaches communicate to others the importance of working together.

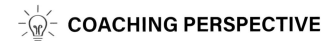

THE POWER OF TEAMWORK

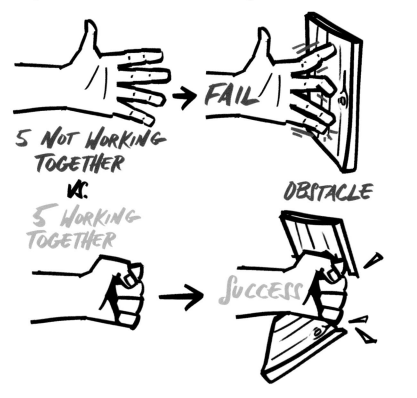

5 NOT WORKING TOGETHER
vs.
5 WORKING TOGETHER

FAIL

OBSTACLE

SUCCESS

h/t Former Duke University Basketball Coach Mike Krzyzewski

What does this mean?

For coaches of team sports, the hand/fist analogy may help communicate to athletes why working together toward a common goal is more effective than working independently.

CHAPTER ⑭

EDUCATION

$$\text{⏻} = \frac{\text{🔨🔧}}{\text{🕐}}$$

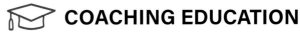

6 AREAS OF EFFECTIVE COACHING

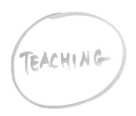 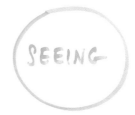 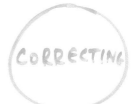

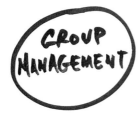 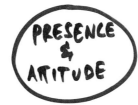 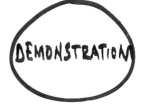

✳ CONTENT KNOWLEDGE

✳ SOCIAL KNOWLEDGE

h/t CrossFit Training & Education (@crossfittraining)

What does this mean?

There are primarily six different areas of coaching:

- Teaching (communicating how to move correctly)
- Seeing (identifying movement efficiencies and faults)
- Correcting (helping athletes improve their movement)
- Group management (leading a group of athletes through a workout)
- Presence and attitude
- Demonstrating

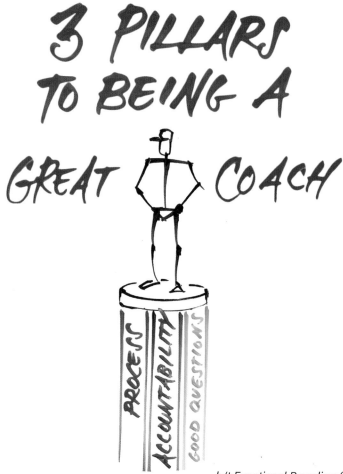

h/t Functional Branding (@functionalbranding)
via Patrick Cummings (@pscummings)

What does this mean?

Process: Great coaches don't just wing it and hope for the best. They have a philosophy, a framework, and systems in place to address multiple situations.

Accountability: Just as iron sharpens iron, great coaches need to be coached by other great coaches.

Good questions: Questions provoke thought that leads to solutions. However, to be able to ask the right questions, the coach must have the corresponding subject knowledge.

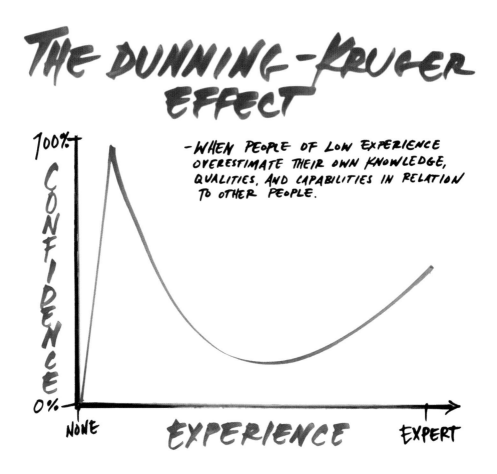

THE DUNNING - KRUGER EFFECT

- WHEN PEOPLE OF LOW EXPERIENCE OVERESTIMATE THEIR OWN KNOWLEDGE, QUALITIES, AND CAPABILITIES IN RELATION TO OTHER PEOPLE.

100%

0%

CONFIDENCE

NONE

EXPERIENCE

EXPERT

What does this mean?

Novices tend to overestimate their knowledge and ability. Their newfound knowledge (however small it may be), ignorance, and lack of experience leads to a spike in confidence, which then leads them to believe that they know everything they need to know about the subject.

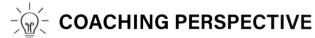
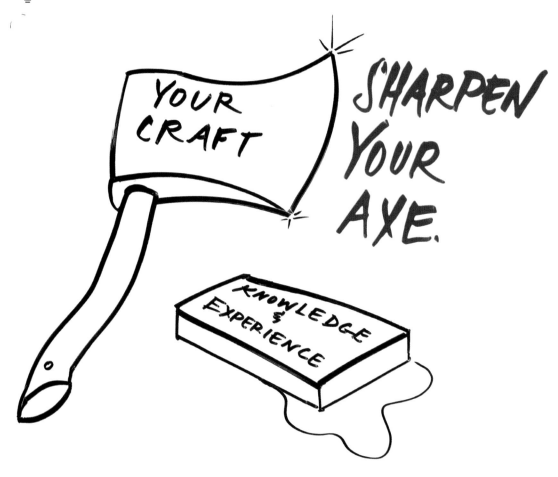

What does this mean?

When productivity and inspiration drop (and they will), take a break. However, understand that during a break, you're not sharpening your axe; you're putting your axe down.

Sharpening the axe is an activity. Take the time and effort to invest in yourself. For example, I took a break to attend a two-day gymnastics course that was packed with knowledge that I could take back to my gym and share on WBD. I was sharpening my axe.

THE IMPORTANCE OF TECHNIQUE

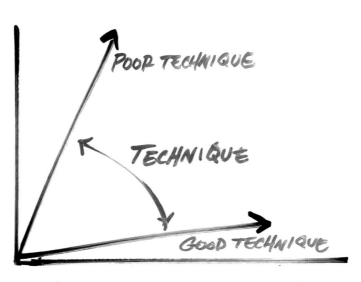

What does this mean?

Technique is the movement or positions used to accomplish a task. The better an athlete's technique is, the less energy they need to use to get a job done. When movement is the subject, technique must be an ongoing focus of the lesson.

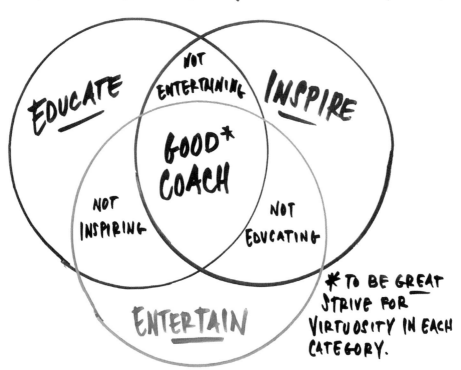

WHAT MAKES A GOOD COACH?

EDUCATE

NOT ENTERTAINING

INSPIRE

GOOD* COACH

NOT INSPIRING

NOT EDUCATING

ENTERTAIN

*TO BE GREAT STRIVE FOR VIRTUOSITY IN EACH CATEGORY.

What does this mean?

Good coaches

- Educate
- Inspire
- Entertain

Good coaches have subject knowledge and a desire to share that knowledge, and they have an even stronger desire to learn more for the primary reason of providing the most value to their athletes. Good coaches have an ability to motivate their athletes so that they are able to push themselves beyond what they would have done on their own. Furthermore, good coaches must be able to get their athletes engaged with the training so that they are excited to show up and work hard. If you strive for these qualities, you'll be on your way to being a good coach.

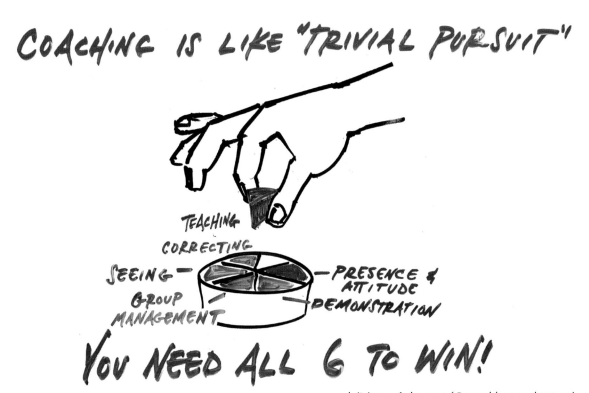

COACHING IS LIKE "TRIVIAL PURSUIT"

TEACHING
CORRECTING
SEEING
GROUP MANAGEMENT
PRESENCE & ATTITUDE
DEMONSTRATION

YOU NEED ALL 6 TO WIN!

h/t Jason Ackerman (@coachjasonackerman)

What does this mean?

Effective coaching is like the board game Trivial Pursuit—relying on one category will get you only so far. You need all six categories to win.

Here are six criteria to be an effective coach:

- Teaching
- Seeing
- Correcting
- Group management
- Demonstration
- Presence and attitude

As a coach, you must push yourself to strengthen your weaknesses, just as you should push your athletes to strengthen theirs. Work on your weaknesses so much that they become your strengths.

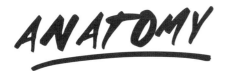

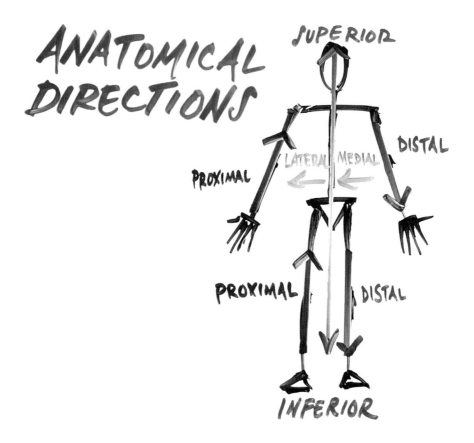

- **Superior:** Higher on the vertical axis
- **Inferior:** Lower on the vertical axis

- **Medial:** Toward midline
- **Lateral:** Away from midline

- **Proximal:** Closer to origin
- **Distal:** Farther from origin

ANATOMICAL MOVEMENT

ANKLE

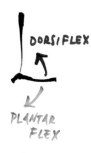

HAND

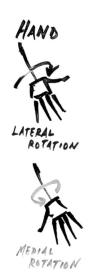

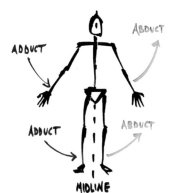

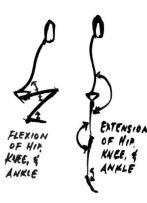

- **Abduction:** Movement away from midline
- **Adduction:** Movement toward midline

- **Flexion:** Decrease the angle of two body parts
- **Extension:** Increase the angle of two body parts

- **Medial rotation:** Rotational movement toward midline
- **Lateral rotation:** Rotational movement away from midline

- **Dorsiflexion:** Flexion of the ankle
- **Plantar flexion:** Extension of the ankle

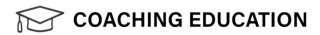
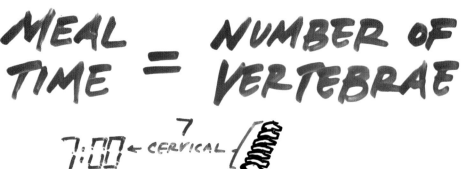

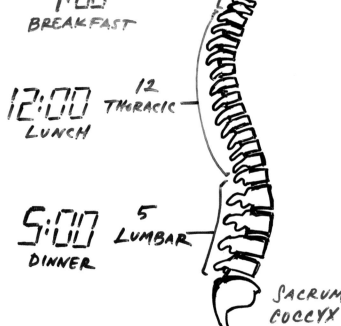

h/t Charlie Cates (@charliecates)

You can use a meal-related mnemonic to remember the number of vertebrae in each section of the spine.

- Breakfast at 7:00 a.m. = 7 cervical vertebrae
- Lunch at 12:00 p.m. = 12 thoracic vertebrae
- Dinner at 5:00 p.m. = 5 lumbar vertebrae

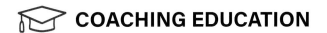
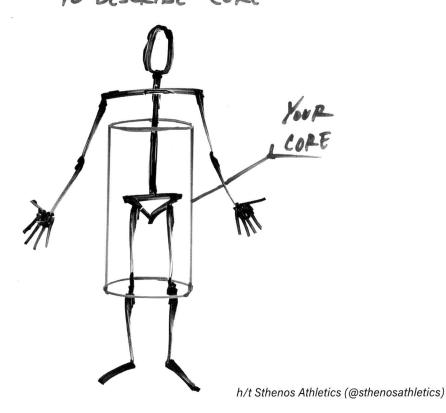

h/t Sthenos Athletics (@sthenosathletics)

What does this mean?

This simple rhyme loosely defines the location of the core.

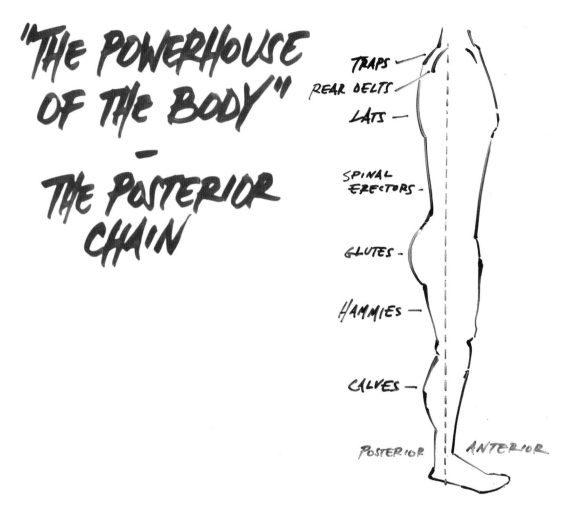

"THE POWERHOUSE OF THE BODY" — THE POSTERIOR CHAIN

TRAPS
REAR DELTS
LATS
SPINAL ERECTORS
GLUTES
HAMMIES
CALVES
POSTERIOR — ANTERIOR

What does this mean?

Commonly referred to as "the powerhouse of the body," the posterior chain is the group of muscles on the back side of the body. This group of muscles works together to perform a long list of movements, including the opening of the hip joint, a requirement in nearly every explosive movement in athletics and conditioning.

Strengthening the posterior chain is crucial not only for sports performance but, more important, for functional movement performed in everyday life. Want to get better at jumping, pushing, pulling, running, squatting, and standing up? Strengthen "the powerhouse of your body": your posterior chain.

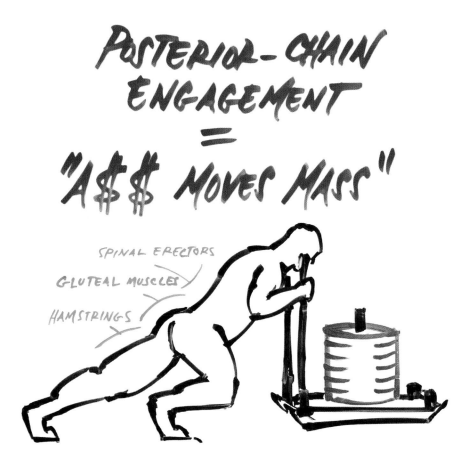

PosterioR-CHAIN
Engagement
=
"A$$ Moves Mass"

SPINAL ERECTORS
GLUTEAL MUSCLES
HAMSTRINGS

h/t CrossFit Training & Education (@crossfittraining)

What does this mean?

This simple rhyme helps explain the power of the posterior chain. When it comes to generating power, the engine of the body is found in the rear.

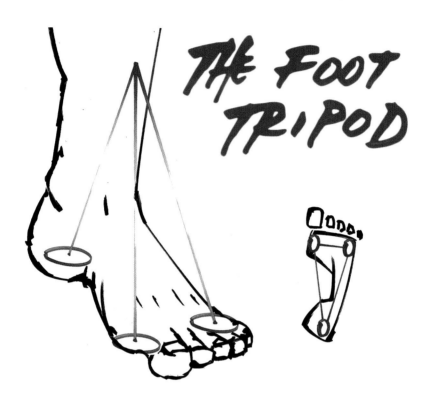

h/t Wil Fleming (@wilfleming)

What does this mean?

The foot tripod refers to three points of contact that the bottom of the foot makes with the ground.

Why?

This term is an easy way to specifically explain the even distribution of weight in the foot. Pushing through the "whole foot (tripod), the whole time" will help the athlete keep balanced even when holding weight.

TEACHING

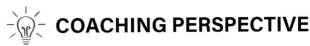 **COACHING PERSPECTIVE**

TECHNICAL LINGO < UNDERSTANDING

INSTEAD OF:	TRY:
TRIPLE EXTENSION	JUMP
EXTERNAL ROTATION	POINT ELBOWS DOWN
ACTIVATE YOUR GLUTES	SQUEEZE YOUR BUTT
CONTRACT YOUR ABDOMINALS	BRACE FOR A PUNCH

h/t Stronghold Mentoring (@strongholdmentoring)

What does this mean?

As a coach, using technical jargon (supine, proximal, superior, etc.) is fine, as long as your athlete understands what you mean.

"Your job is to help people understand, not impress them with your 'super smart' lingo."

—@strongholdmentoring

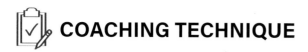 **COACHING TECHNIQUE**

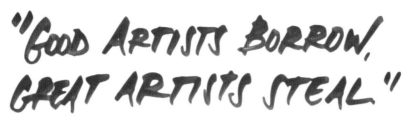

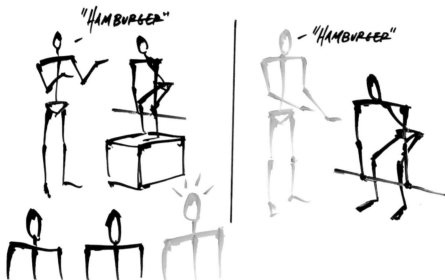

What does this mean?

You may have heard the phrase "art imitates art." The same applies to coaching cues. As coaches are developing their cues, they can borrow from other coaches who have been motivating or inspiring with their coaching techniques. Communicating movement and creating and delivering coaching cues can easily be seen as an art form. Watch the best coaches. Learn from them. Then use what has worked for them on your athletes.

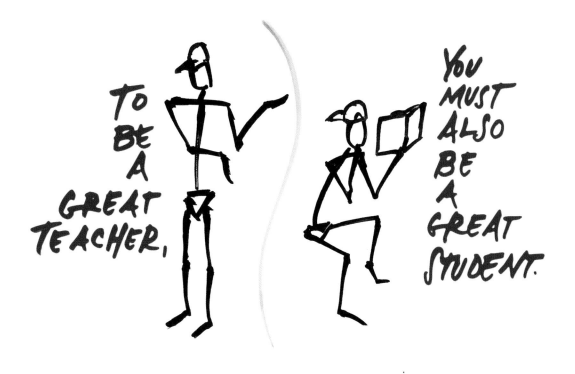

TO BE A GREAT TEACHER,

YOU MUST ALSO BE A GREAT STUDENT.

What does this mean?

Coaches are teachers and distributors of knowledge. To share that knowledge with others, there must be a constant pursuit of education; so great coaches have a passion not only for helping others but also for being students. Always learning. Always growing.

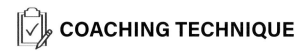

COACHING TECHNIQUE

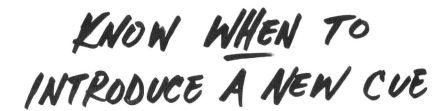

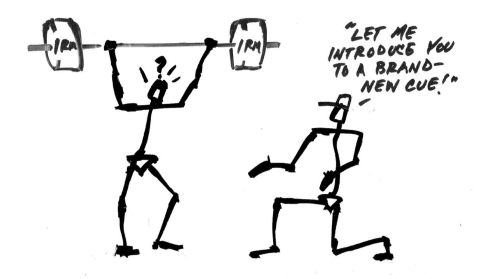

What does this mean?

The optimal time to introduce a new cue is during the warm-up and light working sets. This is the best setting for the athlete to take in a new concept while moving a weight that is still easy for them.

The heavier the weight is or the higher the intensity of the setting (mid-WOD), the higher the likelihood the athlete will get distracted or lose focus if they are also engaged in the task of comprehending a new cue.

This isn't to say that introducing a new cue when the athlete is under high stress won't work. It just isn't the best time to do it.

SEEING

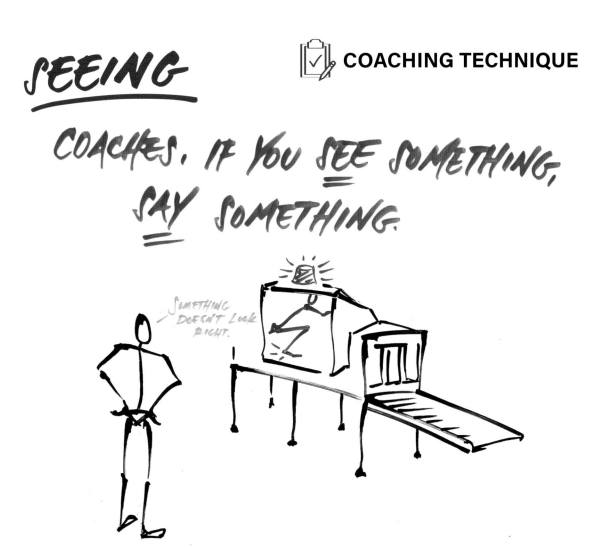

COACHES. IF YOU SEE SOMETHING, SAY SOMETHING.

SOMETHING DOESN'T LOOK RIGHT.

What does this mean?

A coach's job is simply to improve the performance of your athlete. If you see something that may help them (spoiler alert: there is *always* something), it is your job to tell them. It's like the national campaign to raise public awareness of homeland security: If you see something, say something!

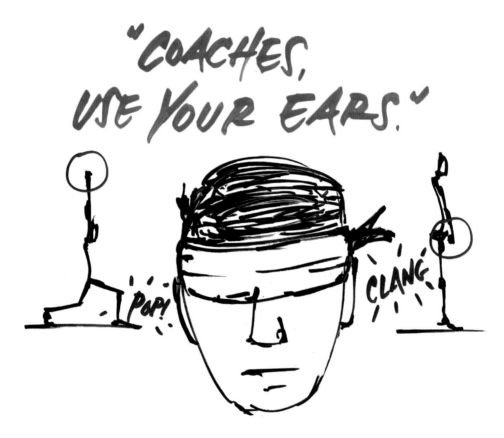

What does this mean?

Coaches are tasked with helping athletes improve. It goes without saying that each athlete moves differently and has their own strengths and weaknesses.

Following a listening:talking ratio of 2:1 helps coaches better understand how to address athletes' individual differences. While coaching an individual or a group, discipline yourself to listen and observe twice as much as you talk.

> "We have two ears, and one mouth and we should use them proportionally."
>
> **—SUSAN CAIN**

CORRECTING

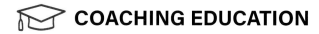

"BLANK YOUR BLANK"

VERBAL CUEING BASICS

FLEX YOUR QUADS

SQUEEZE YOUR GLUTES

STRAIGHTEN YOUR KNEES

What does this mean?

Think of this as "Verbal Cueing for Beginners." Cues should be specific, actionable, and short. One of the best ways to give cues is to follow the template "_____ your _____." This will help you keep cues straightforward and easy to understand.

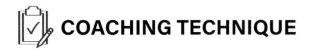
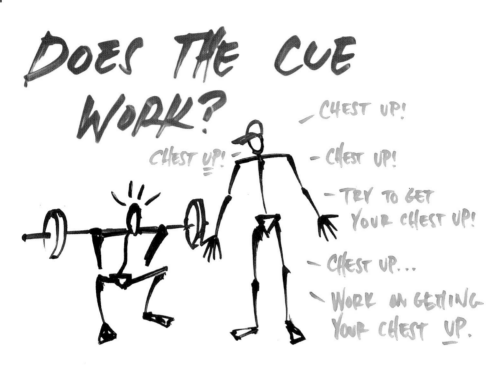

What does this mean?

Fight the urge to say the same cue over and over again, especially if it doesn't work. Coaches need to have a wide repertoire of methods to communicate proper movement. If a verbal cue doesn't work, try a tactile cue. If that doesn't work, try a visual cue. Insanity is doing the same thing over and over again and expecting a different result. Don't be an insane coach!

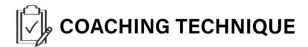
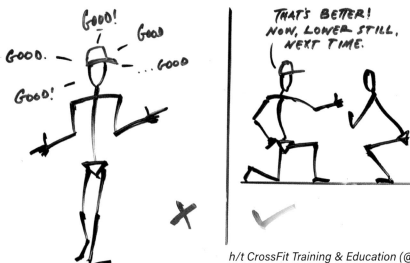

h/t CrossFit Training & Education (@crossfittraining)
L2 Certificate Course Training Guide

What does this mean?

It's very easy to try to be encouraging to your athlete and simply say "good" each time they move, *even if* the movement wasn't good. Instead of falling into this habit, provide your athletes with some valuable feedback. How can their movement be better (there is always something that can be improved)? After you provide a cue, is their movement the same, better, or worse?

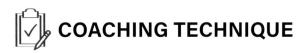

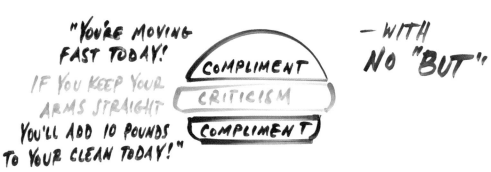

TRY SERVING A
"CRITICISM SANDWICH"

"YOU'RE MOVING FAST TODAY!

IF YOU KEEP YOUR ARMS STRAIGHT

YOU'LL ADD 10 POUNDS TO YOUR CLEAN TODAY!"

COMPLIMENT
CRITICISM
COMPLIMENT

— WITH NO "BUT"

h/t "Coaching the Positive" by Ben Bergeron in The CrossFit Journal

When?

If an athlete is getting frustrated with a movement, try serving a compliment sandwich when providing feedback.

Why?

Bookend your constructive criticism with positive remarks. The balance of this technique may help the athlete stay encouraged, especially when they feel frustrated.

> *"Encourage with enthusiasm. That's your job, and it's the responsibility of the coach. It's a small critique that goes a long way."*

—BEN BERGERON

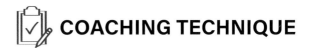

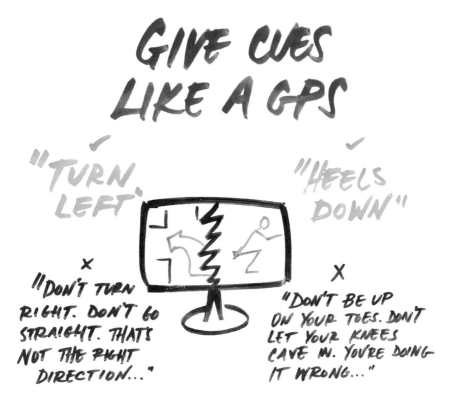

h/t Ben Bergeron (@benbergeron)

What does this mean?

Keep cues direct, short, and actionable, like the directions from a GPS app.

How a GPS *doesn't* work:

- "Go down the street, slow down around the curve, then turn right, then..."
- "Don't turn left. Don't turn left. Don't turn left."

How a GPS *does* work:

- "Turn left now."
- "Keep straight for 50 miles."

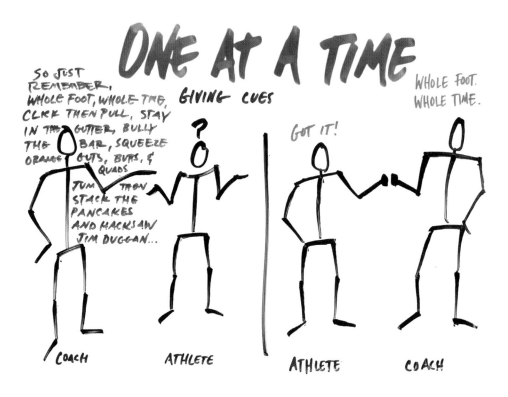

What does this mean?

Verbal cues, especially when short, specific, and actionable, can be extremely effective for communicating movement. I encourage you to focus on one thing at a time, especially when working with novice athletes.

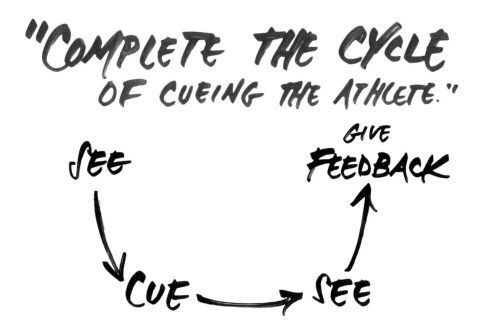

"COMPLETE THE CYCLE OF CUEING THE ATHLETE."

SEE → CUE → SEE → GIVE FEEDBACK

h/t Steve Haydock (@stevehaydock)

What does this mean?

The process of cueing the athlete doesn't stop with simply providing the cue:

- Watch the athlete move.
- Provide a cue to improve the movement.
- Watch the athlete move again.
- Provide feedback. Was the next attempt the same, better, or worse?

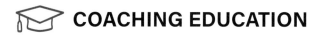
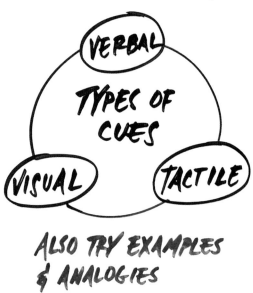

"AN EFFECTIVE CUE IS ONE THAT WORKS."

TYPES OF CUES

VERBAL

VISUAL

TACTILE

ALSO TRY EXAMPLES & ANALOGIES

What does this mean?

Cues are *always* athlete dependent. What works for one person may not work for another. The more cues you have in your mental toolbox, the more likely you will be able to communicate a correction.

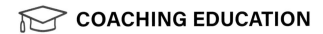
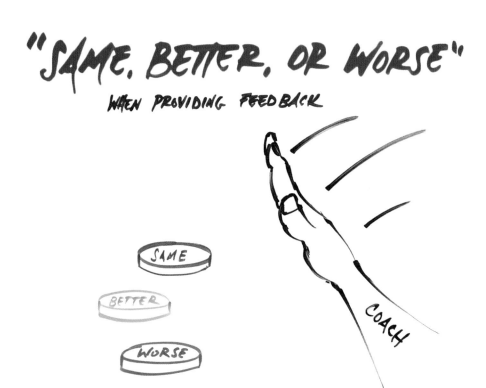

h/t CrossFit Training & Education (@crossfittraining)
L2 Certificate Course Training Guide

When?

Use this concept to assess cues' effectiveness and provide feedback to athletes.

What does this mean?

A trainer's job is to let the athlete know if the movement was the same, better, or worse than the last time they performed that movement. Providing no response is unacceptable. There is always an opportunity for feedback.

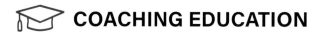
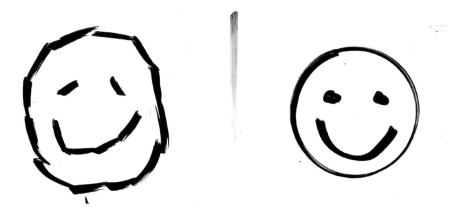

What does this mean?

In these two drawings, the same relative message is communicated. However, one uses far fewer lines.

Imagine the lines of a drawing are like words when coaching. Chuck Carswell reminds us that cues should be actionable, effective, and *short*.

Of course, this skill takes time to develop, but it's worth the effort not to lose your athlete with long, complex descriptions. Find ways to communicate the same message with fewer words.

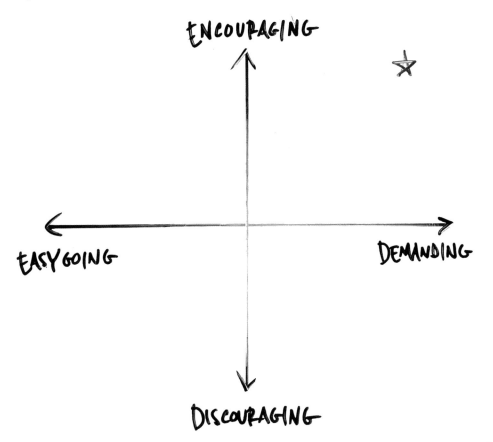

PRESENCE & ATTITUDE

THE APPROACH OF A GOOD COACH

ENCOURAGING

EASYGOING

DEMANDING

DISCOURAGING

h/t Wil Fleming (@wilfleming)

What does this mean?

A good coach is 100% encouraging *and* 100% demanding. Always see the best possible outcome for your athlete *and* help them understand the work it will take to get there.

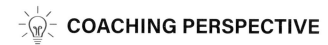
P.R. I.D.E.

PERSONAL RESPONSIBILITY IN DAILY EXCELLENCE

h/t Ben Bergeron (@benbergeron)

What does this mean?

Pride can be seen as a double-edged sword. The two sides represent the good and bad that can come from having pride.

Being *too* proud leads to having an ego, which can keep a person from being their best self. However, if a person takes pride in their efforts, values, and conduct, it can lead them to reach their goals.

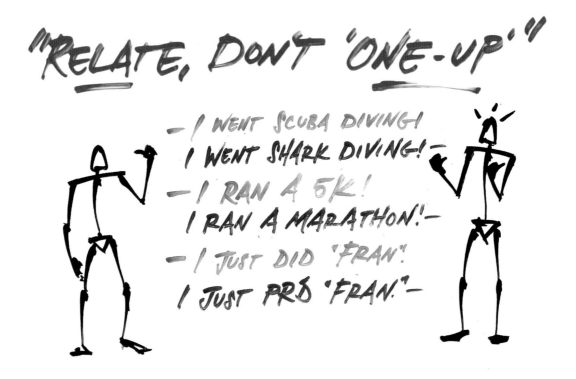

"RELATE, DON'T 'ONE-UP'"

- I WENT SCUBA DIVING!
- I WENT SHARK DIVING!
- I RAN A 5K!
- I RAN A MARATHON!
- I JUST DID "FRAN".
- I JUST PR'd "FRAN."

h/t Ben Bergeron (@benbergeron) and Patrick Cummings (@pscummings)

What does this mean?

Coaches want to connect with people, but that doesn't mean they need to try to impress them with accomplishments. Instead of "one-upping" another person, simply ask them a few more questions about *their* experience. That type of interaction will go much further in developing relationships.

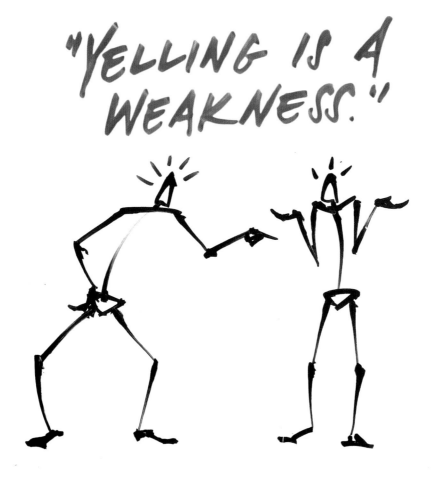

"YELLING IS A WEAKNESS."

h/t Jocko Willink (@jockowillink)

What does this mean?

Have you ever been yelled at by someone in a leadership position and thought, "Wow, I'm very impressed with how they are handling this situation"? Probably not.

If you have to yell as a leader, the unfortunate situation you're in is likely your fault. When you are yelling at someone, their respect for you is declining as you are demonstrating your inability to control your emotions and make the right decisions that a leader should be able to make. Yelling is a weakness. Don't do it.

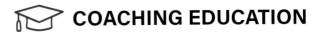

"EATING WHILE COACHING"

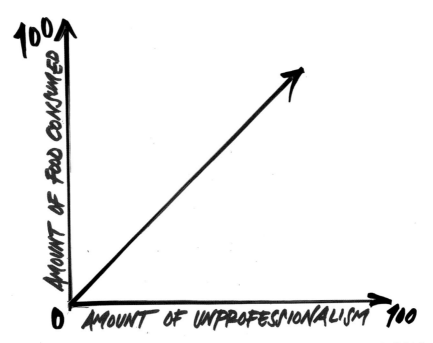

h/t Matt DellaValle (@mdv_fit)

What does this mean?

The bigger the serving, the bigger the error. In a world where professionalism matters (the fitness industry), this should not happen. Don't eat while you are coaching.

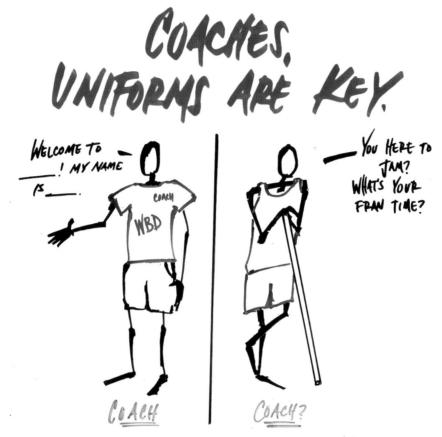

h/t Jason Fernandez (@jfern3)

What does this mean?

A coach needs to look the part to help athletes, particularly walk-ins, know who is coaching.

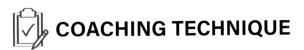
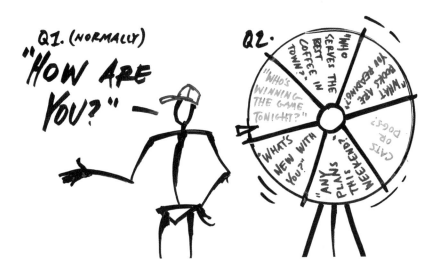

h/t Chuck Carswell via James Hobart (@jameshobart)

What does this mean?

Coaches often ask, "How are you?" But you shouldn't stop there. Ask a second question about what your athlete is up to. It's not an interrogation. Asking questions helps you get a better understanding of who they are and how you can relate to them.

"COACH THE POSITIVE."

THE POWER OF WORDS

- NEGATIVE -	- POSITIVE -
"I CAN'T BELIEVE HOW FAST YOU DID THAT!" →	"YOU WERE SO FAST TODAY. KEEP IT UP!"
"YOU NEED TO WORK ON YOUR GYMNASTICS" →	"W/ YOUR WORK ETHIC, YOU'RE GOING TO GET BETTER AT GYMNASTICS"
"DON'T PUT THE BAR DOWN!" →	"BIG SET, HERE!"

h/t Ben Bergeron (@benbergeron)

What does this mean?

Words have power and greatly influence athletes and their performance. What a coach tells an athlete can get replayed in their mind over and over until it is a self-fulfilling prophecy. Understand that words lead to thoughts, thoughts lead to action, actions lead to habits, and habits can determine an outcome. Use your words for good!

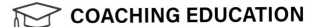

5 REASONS WHY COACHES SHOULD LEAD WARM-UPS

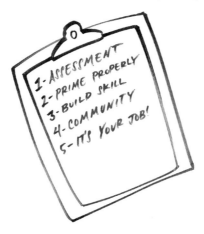

1 - ASSESSMENT
2 - PRIME PROPERLY
3 - BUILD SKILL
4 - COMMUNITY
5 - IT'S YOUR JOB!

What does this mean?

The benefits of warming up are no secret, but the importance of this time being led by a coach should also be well understood.

- **Assessment:** The warm-up provides the coach with the crucial time to observe the quality of movement of their athlete(s) and properly cue them (verbal, visual, and tactile) prior to adding weight to a movement.

- **Prime properly:** The coach should know the workout, including the intended stimulus and targeted muscle groups/energy systems, better than anyone. The warm-up provides the coach a time to share this info and explain the tailoring of the movements.

- **Build skill:** Virtuosity is performing the common uncommonly well. The warm-up provides the coach a time to build in skill work at a point when the athlete is fresh and unfatigued.

- **Community:** Warm-up time allows the coach time to interact with the athlete(s) (and athletes with each other) prior to "3-2-1-go!"

- **It's your job:** Your athlete(s) should get the best from you from the moment they check in to after class is over (and then some).

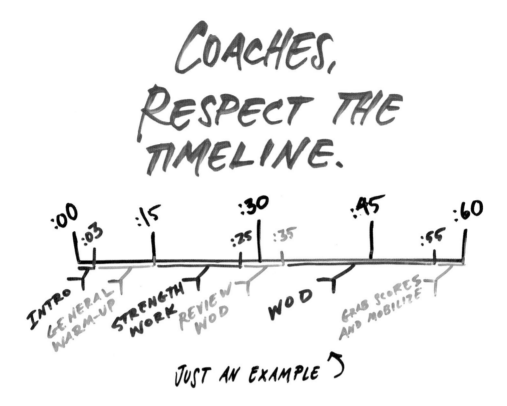

What does this mean?

Accuracy is one of the ten general physical skills in CrossFit. This also applies to a coach's class time management. Running over and finishing early are both signs of poor planning. Respect your athletes' time and money and plan ahead.

"PUT AWAY WHATEVER YOU USE."

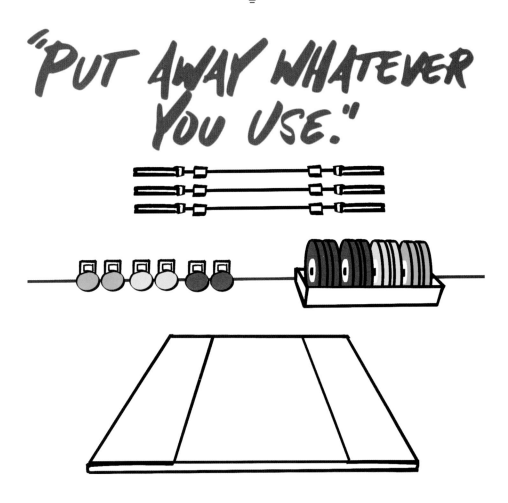

What does this mean?

Putting things away after you use them is a common life skill that you were likely taught in kindergarten, and it is one of the most important unwritten rules of any gym. If the person before you didn't put it away correctly, be the better person and do it right. A clean gym is organized and safe.

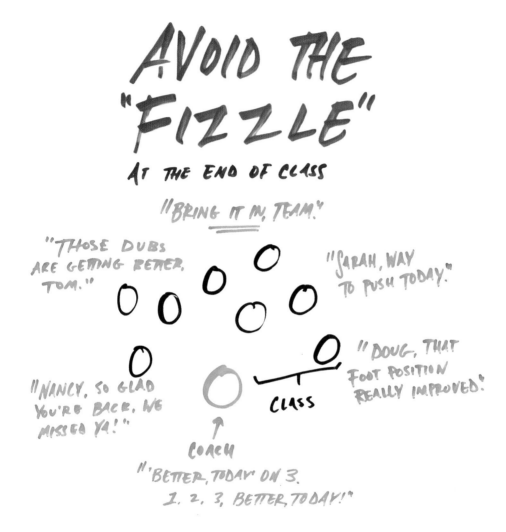

AVOID THE "FIZZLE"

AT THE END OF CLASS

"BRING IT IN, TEAM."

"THOSE DUBS ARE GETTING BETTER, TOM."

"SARAH, WAY TO PUSH TODAY."

"DOUG, THAT FOOT POSITION REALLY IMPROVED!"

"NANCY, SO GLAD YOU'RE BACK. WE MISSED YA!"

CLASS

COACH

"'BETTER, TODAY' ON 3. 1. 2. 3. BETTER, TODAY!"

What does this mean?

Whether you're a coach or an athlete, you've likely experienced the fizzle that can happen at the end of class. The last person finishes the workout, the timer ends, and then everyone puts their equipment away and heads off. The first 59 minutes had great energy, and then it...fizzles out.

My suggestion is that coaches bring the athletes in, hand out some encouragement, and use that last minute to wrap things up. Build your community and coach like you mean it.

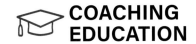
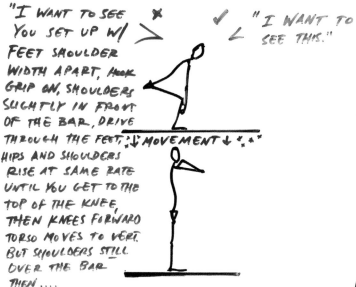

MINIMIZE YOUR TALKING WHILE YOU'RE DEMOING

"I WANT TO SEE YOU SET UP W/ FEET SHOULDER WIDTH APART, HOOK GRIP ON, SHOULDERS SLIGHTLY IN FRONT OF THE BAR, DRIVE THROUGH THE FEET, HIPS AND SHOULDERS RISE AT SAME RATE UNTIL YOU GET TO THE TOP OF THE KNEE, THEN KNEES FORWARD TORSO MOVES TO VERT. BUT SHOULDERS STILL OVER THE BAR THEN ....

↓ MOVEMENT ↓

✓ "I WANT TO SEE THIS."

h/t Chuck Carswell

What does this mean?

Keep talking to a minimum as you demonstrate a movement. Keep your instruction short and simple, like this:

"You are here." [START POSITION]

"What I want to see is this."
[MOVEMENT]

Why?

When you talk and demo, you're going to make a mistake.

Need more help?

For more information, see "Minimize Talking While Demonstrating with Chuck Carswell" at www.youtube.com/watch?v=M9jWUj1nK90.

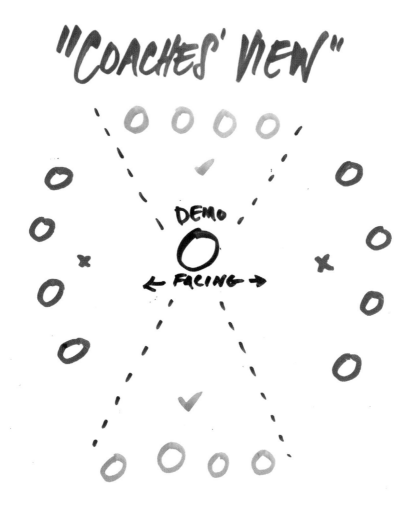

What does this mean?

When coaching, it's important to consider your athlete when demonstrating a movement.

There is a reason why judges are positioned to the side of gymnasts and CrossFit Games competitors. It's the same reason why every post from @hookgrip shows the side view of an Olympic lifter. That's where all the good stuff is.

When demoing, encourage your athletes to stand in the "coaches' view"—the view *you* take to see how your athletes move. This should help them further understand your instruction.

STRENGTH TRAINING BASICS

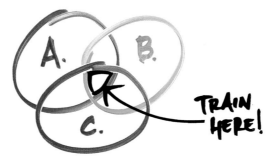

A: REASONABLE - "START TOO LIGHT"
B: CONSISTENT - "DON'T MISS WORKOUTS"
C: IMPROVEMENT - "TAKE SMALL STEPS"

h/t James Clear (@jamesclear)

What does this mean?

Simplify your approach and focus on the fundamentals, not the details:

- **Start light:** Lighter weights allow the lifter to establish proper movement patterns. As the weight gets heavier, form becomes exponentially more important.

- **Be consistent:** Progress is created from sustained and sensible effort.

- **Take small steps:** The shorter the steps, the longer the journey.

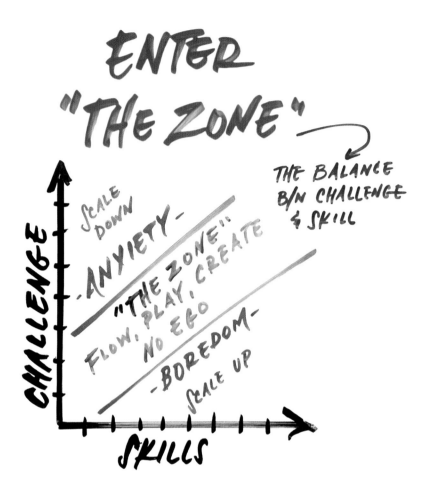

What does this mean?

The zone is a state of flow—a state of concentration or complete absorption in an activity.

The creator of the illustrated model, psychologist Mihaly Csikszentmihalyi, describes the zone as "being completely involved in an activity for its own sake. The ego falls away."

How do you create an opportunity for "the zone" within your training? Scale accordingly. When the activity is too challenging, scale down. When the activity is too easy, scale up. Within that sweet spot between challenge and skills, you'll find your zone.

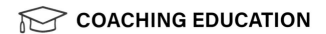
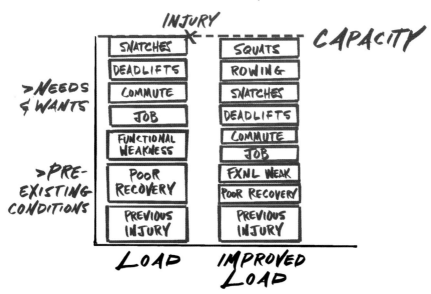

h/t Active Life Professional (@activelifeprofessional)
via Dr. Sean Pastuch (@drseanpastuch)

What does this mean?

Just like it's rarely the last point that wins the game, it's rarely the last rep that is the cause of injury.

Injury happens when load exceeds capacity:

- LOAD = preexisting conditions + needs and wants
- CAPACITY = injury threshold

How can athletes avoid injury?

First, decrease preexisting conditions:

- Improve recovery
- Improve weaknesses

Second, increase capacity (Athlete Hierarchy of Needs):

- Flexibility
- Mobility
- Strength balance
- Volume and recovery balance
- Skill/motor control

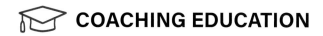
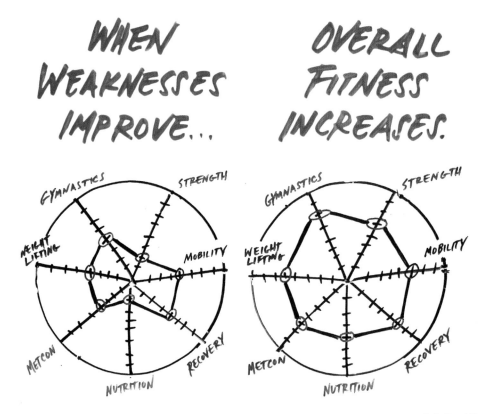

h/t @eddiesmethod

What does this mean?

By improving capacity in the weak areas, overall fitness continues to increase.

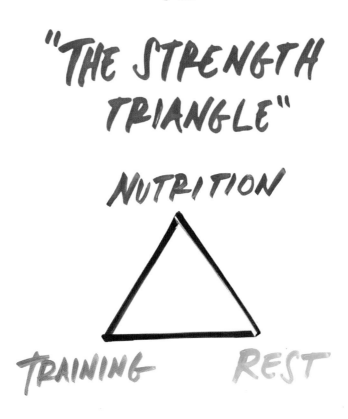

"THE STRENGTH TRIANGLE"

NUTRITION

TRAINING   REST

h/t Bill Starr

What does this mean?

There are three equal sides to the strength triangle: training, nutrition, and rest. Each of these is just as important as the others and unique to the individual.

ACKNOWLEDGMENTS

Thank you to my wife, Ali, for always being supportive and encouraging of this passion project of mine. I believe balance is crucial in any successful partnership. You are the left brain to my right brain. When I had a vision for Whiteboard Daily, you helped me see details that I overlooked and worked with me to create a plan and follow through to accomplish my goals. Thank you for being my partner with this and in life.

Thank you to my parents, Jim and Kay, for always being supportive of me and encouraging me to be creative. I've always known I had an artistic side, thanks to you, but never knew how I could express it. Thank you for always enthusiastically cheering me on.

Thank you to my brothers, Erik and Kurt, for their inspiration as they pursue their own creative endeavors. I'm amazed at how both of you have grown to be incredible artists, and how all three of us have developed our skills to pursue our unique passions.

To Greg Everett, Catalyst Athletics: You have been a massive inspiration for me. The amount of instructional content you have shared throughout your coaching career can arguably be considered one of the most valuable contributions to the world of Olympic weightlifting. I can't thank you enough for all that you have taught me.

To Sevan Mattosian: CrossFit was an integral part of my coaching journey. Your friendship and our workouts in Berkeley played a massive role in me learning and teaching others all that I could.

To Wil Fleming, 1K Weightlifting: Wil, your coaching introduced me to cues and perspectives that inspired me to create this book. You are a phenomenal coach, and I'm honored to be able to call you a friend.

To Mike Burgener, Burgener Strength: A sign of a great coach is how they can simplify complex movements, and few movements are more complex than the snatch, clean, and jerk. Your keen ability to do this has inspired me to do the same.

To Danny Lehr, Caffeine & Kilos: I have always admired how you and Dean have created such a successful lifestyle brand, especially one that has made such an impact on the fitness community. Thank you for collaborating with WBD on all of our past projects, and those in the future.

To Michael Lian, Get RX'd: When Whiteboard Daily was in its early stages, you saw the value and potential of what WBD had to offer—enough to be a generous and sole sponsor of WBD. Thank you for believing in my mission.

To Chuck Bennington, The Gymnastics Course: When I had just started WBD, I reached out to a ton of subject matter experts within the CrossFit world. You were the very first not only to respond but to work with me to help WBD to the next level.

To Lynden Reder, Velaasa: Thank you for partnering on the WBD x Velaasa Strake weightlifting shoes. I consider them works of art, and they are currently (and always will be) displayed in a case in my office.

To Dylan Tellem, AbMat: Thank you for collaborating on the WBD x AbMat Crash Cushions. You guys are truly innovators within the fitness industry and have only just begun improving the products that people use to exercise.

To Jason Ackerman, Best Hour of Their Day: Thank you for collaborating with me on the WBD Podcast and the very first WBD e-book. Your subject knowledge expertise, not only in the realm of fitness but even more so in business development, helped me take WBD to the next level.

To Aaron James, CrossFit MANA: Thank you for inspiring me to be a coach and providing an opportunity for me to do so. The New Zealand flag that carries the well-wishes of the MANA whanau is proudly displayed in my office.

To Slater Coe, Derby City CrossFit: Thank you for being my longest CrossFit friend and for giving me the opportunity to coach at your world-class facility.

To Jared Byczko and Peter Brasovan, Myriad Health & Fitness: Thank you for giving me an opportunity to pursue my passion and an outlet to share my knowledge with others.

To Glen Cordoza: Thank you for seeing the value in WBD and reaching out to me to make this dream of mine a reality.

To Susan Lloyd, Pam Mourouzis, Charlotte Kughen, Kat Lannom, Justin-Aaron Velasco, Lance Freimuth, and the rest of the Victory Belt Publishing team: If it weren't for you, this book would not have been a reality. No question. Thank you for believing in this book, your hard work, and your expertise to make this project a success.

FAN PHOTOS

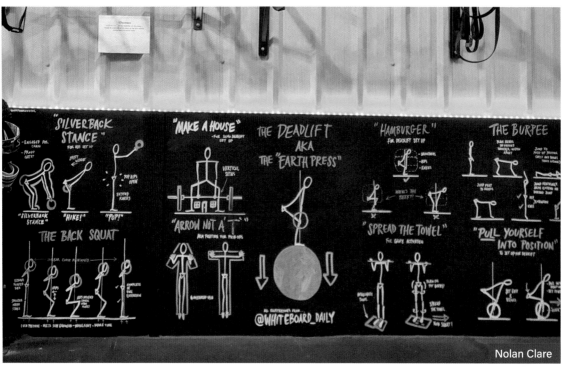

Nolan Clare

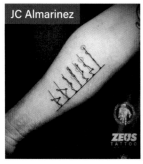

JC Almarinez

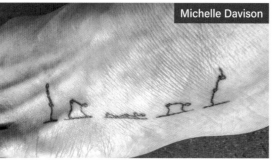

Michelle Davison

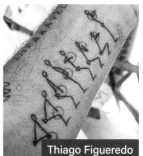

Thiago Figueredo

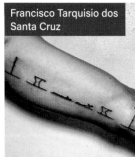

Francisco Tarquisio dos Santa Cruz

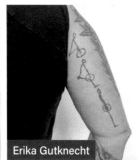

Erika Gutknecht

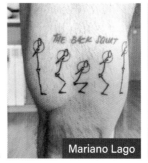

Mariano Lago

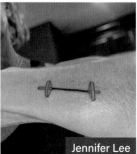

Jennifer Lee

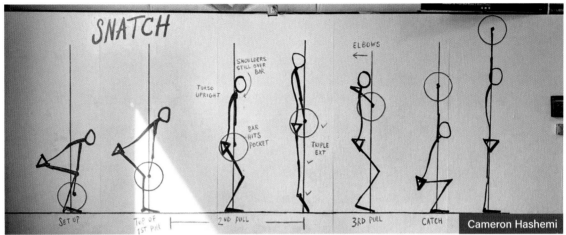
SNATCH

SHOULDERS STILL OVER BAR

TORSO UPRIGHT

BAR HITS POCKET

ELBOWS

TRIPLE EXT

SET UP | TOP OF 1ST PULL | 2ND PULL | 3RD PULL | CATCH

Cameron Hashemi

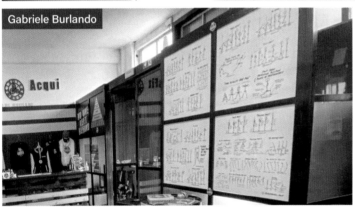
Gabriele Burlando

Acqui

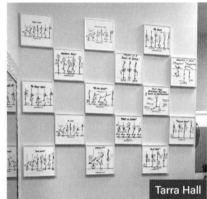
Tarra Hall

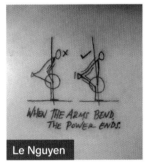
WHEN THE ARMS BEND THE POWER ENDS.

Le Nguyen

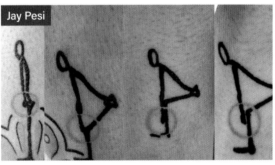
Jay Pesi

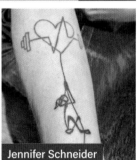
Jennifer Schneider

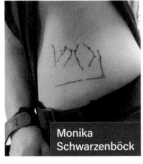
Monika Schwarzenböck

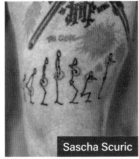
Sascha Scuric

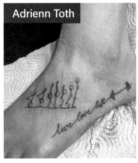
Adrienn Toth

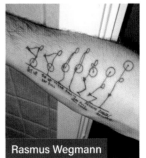
Rasmus Wegmann

TITLE INDEX

Numbers

1:2, 220
3 Pillars to Being a Great Coach, 346
3-Position Clean, 130
3 S's, The, 318
5 Not 3, 124
5 Reasons Why Coaches Should Lead
    Warm-Ups, 383
5 Reasons to Wrap Your Thumb Around
    the Bar, 239
6 Areas of Effective Coaching, 345

A

Air Squat, The, 9
All Reps Matter, 266
Aluminum Can, 236
Amsterdam, 221
Anatomical Directions, 352
Anatomical Movement, 353
Anatomy of a Kettlebell, 181
Approach of a Good Coach, The, 375
Are You a Patient Lifter?, 151
Area of the Base, The, 178
Arms Are Ropes, 140
Arnold Palmer, 78
Arrow Not a T, 62
Ask a Second Question, 381
Ass Moves Mass, 357
Avoid the Fizzle, 386
Avoid the Stripper Booty Error, 97

B

Back Squat, 20
Bad Cheerleader Jump, 46
Bar Is Pivot Point, 159
Bar Speed Builds, 138
Barbell Is a Road Map, 240
Barbell Over Midfoot, 257
Be a Barrel, Not an Hourglass, 232
Be a Leaf Spring, 40
Be a Thermostat, Not a Thermometer,
    291
Be the Arrow, Not the Bow, 185
Before You Master the Barbell, You Must
    First Master the PVC Pipe, 288
Being Comfortable with Being
    Uncomfortable, 295

Bend and Snap, The, 189
Better Start = Better Finish, 267
Big Five, The, 10
Blank Your Blank, 365
Blot out the Sun, 16
Board Between Your Feet, 123
Books Are the Training Weights of the
    Mind, 308
Boss vs. Leader, 283
Break Before You Are Broken, 312
Break the Band, 313
Breathe Like a Crocodile, 233
Brush, Not a Bang, A, 144
Brush Up Your Shirt, 145
Bucket of Water, 258
Butterfly Pull-Up, The, 59

C

Cheat Code, 268
Chest Up, Hips Down, 99
Chest Up into the Bar, 163
Clean, The, 131
Click-Click, Boom!, 164
Close the Window, 70
Coach the Positive, 382
Coaches' View, 388
Coaching Is Like Trivial Pursuit, 351
Comfort→Fear→Learn→Grow, 319
Complete the Cycle of Cueing the
    Athlete, 371
Consistency Is King, 320
Copy Machine, 269
Create a Wedge, 80

D

Deadlift, 77
Deadlift Wiggle, The, 81
Dip, Drive, Punch, 196
Do Not Move the Barbell, 82
Do What You Can with What You Have,
    321
Does the Cue Work?, 366
Don't Be Dumbo, 272
Don't Be a Good Guy, 367
Don't Be a Jerk, 143
Don't Be a Pecker, 67
Don't Count the Days, 303

Don't Forget the Simple Things, 333
Don't Hit the Glass Wall, 194
Don't Rush Your Setup, 271
Don't Skip Stair Steps, 45
Down Like a Rock, Up Like a Rocket,
    114
Drinking Bird, 191
Drive the Elbows Up! , 26
Drive Off Your Knees, 74
Drive the Triangle Straight Up!, 24
Dunning-Kruger Effect, The, 347

E

Earth Press, The, 98
Eating While Coaching, 379
Effective Cue Is One That Works, An,
    372
Elbow Pits Forward, 63
Elbows Above Hands, 146
Elbows Are Lasers, 27
Elbows Drive High and Back, 156
Elbows Out, 141
Elevator Shaft, 113
Enter the Zone, 390
Extend Before You Bend, 157
Eyes on the Horizon, 142

F

F-F-F: Front Foot First, 125
Fall into Pike, 47
Falling Angle, The, 208
Feel Heavy in Your Hands, 83
Feet Are Talons, 22
Feet in a Bucket, 48
Find Your Gear, 273
Find Your Rhythm, 314
Finish the Pull, 147
Finish the Pull 2, 148
Flashlight on Top of Head, 112
Flexibility Versus Mobility, 224
Focus on the Negative, 84
Foot Forward, Hips Back, 33
Foot Is a Bumper Plate, 165
Foot Tripod, The, 358
Force Curve, 216
Four Pillars of Trust, The, 340–341
Frankenstein Squat, The, 34

Front Rack Clock Face, 28
Front Rack Is a Launchpad, 110
Front Rack Triangles of Support, The, 111
Front Squat, The, 25

G

Get Tall Before You Get Small, 160
Give Cues Like a GPS, 369
Gnat's Ass, 172
Go Underwater, 234
Good Artists Borrow, Great Artists Steal, 360
Grip the Ground, 242
Grip the Handle Like You're Holding Two Birds, 219
Grocery Bag/Car Door, 12

H

Half a Heart, 158
Hamburger, 86
Hammer a Fresh Nail, 206
Hand Is Like a J-Cup, 243
Hand on Forehead to Find Crown, 39
Handstand Push-Ups, 37
Hang Position, 129
Hang Power Clean, 133
Have a Blue-Collar Mentality, 296
Have a Short-Term Memory, 302
Hay Is in the Barn, The, 298
Hear Your Feet, 166
Hierarchy of Gravity's Effect on Movement, The, 207
Hierarchy of Joint Health, 226
High & Tight, 186
High Inside Pitch, 49
Higher Your Desire for Success, the Fewer Choices You Have, The, 297
Hike, Hinge, Root, Float, 182
Hike the Kettlebell, 183
Hip Hinge = Bow & Arrow, 203
Hips Play Chicken with the Kettlebell, 187
How Does Injury Happen: Load vs. Capacity, 391
How Important Is Breathwork?, 264
How Important Is Diaphragmatic Breathing?, 265
How You Lift > How Much You Lift, 284
Human Body Is a Wheel, 205
Hungry Butt, 192

I

I Never Lose. I Either Win or Learn, 299
Identifying a Movement Issue, 225
If You Cheat, Your Coach Noticed, 285
If You See Something, Say Something, 363
Ignite Your Lift, 139
Importance of Technique, The, 349
Inaction Costs More Than Action, 322
It's Muscle Up, Not Muscle Forward, 56

J

Jerk, The, 103
Jump Hard, Land Hard, 168
Jump Hard, Not High, 167
Jump Up, Shrug Down, 161
Just Because You Can Add Weight/ Momentum Doesn't Mean You Should, 286

K

K2E Rope Climb, 71
Karate Chop and Flex for False Grip on Rings, 244
Keep It Between the Bolts, 217
Keep Your Bucket Full, 334
Kettlebell Windmill, The, 199
Kipping Ring Muscle-Up, 50
Know When to Introduce a New Cue, 362
Knuckles on Top, 246
Knuckles to the Floor, Not the Door!, 245

L

Last Reps Mirror First Reps, 270
Launch Position, The, 126
Leaders L.E.A.D., 293
Leave Some Gas in the Tank, 315
Leave Your Ego at the Door, 287
Leave Your Fingerprints on the Barbell, 241
Less Hump, More Jump!, 149
Let the Weight Settle, 274
Line Through Bar, Hip, Ankle, 115
Listen to Your Body, 335
Load, Explode, Punch, 109
Loose Hands, 116

M

Make a Foot Tent, 14
Make a House, 100
Make a Mountain, 200
Make a Mountain of Sand Between Your Feet, 87
Make Gecko Hands, 247
Marble on Your Knee, 17
Martini Glass, Not Wine Glass, 30
Meal Time = Number of Vertebrae, 354
Meet the Bar, 169
Micro Goals Lead to Major Goals, 323
Minimize Your Talking While You're Demoing, 387
Mobility Leads to Strength, 223
Moon the Crowd, 190
Move with a Purpose, 280
Movement Hierarchies Relative to Mobility Demands, 227–229
Movement Is the Best Medicine, 307
Muted Hip, 261
My Technique Is Better with a Little Weight on the Bar, 311

N

Nipples to Knees, 360 Degrees, 355
No Angles, 51
No Leaning, No Sitting, No Noise, 300
Nose Knows: 5 Reasons for Nasal Breathing, The, 265

O

Oly Mechanics Hierarchy, 177
One at a Time, 370
Only Two Shapes, 52
Open Two Books, 88
Overhead Pass, 69
Overhead Squat, 29
Own Your Position, 259

P–Q

Patience!, 150
Peace Fingers, 248
Pistol Squat, The, 32
Plane on the Runway, 152
Poor Recovery Catches Up to You, 337
Power Clean, 132
Power Snatch, 135
Power of Teamwork, The, 343
Powerhouse of the Body, The, 356
PR Wheel, The, 325
Practice, 326
Press in Clean, 134
Press in Snatch, 137
Press in Split, 105

P.R.I.D.E., 376

Proper Preparation Prevents Poor Performance, 327

Proud Chest, 89

Pull the Bar Apart, 249

Pull the Slack Out, 90

Pull Your Elbows Down, 60

Pull Yourself into Position, 91

Pull-Over, The, 58

Pull-Up Grip→Kettlebell Grip, 250

Punch That Mofo Really Hard, 170

Punch the Plywood, 119

Punch the Sky, 118

Push the Earth Away, for deadlift, 92

Push the Earth Away, for push-ups, 64

Push-up, The, 61

Put Away Whatever You Use, 385

Put Down Your Ego to Pick Up the Bar, 289

Put Your Shoulder Blades in Your Back Pocket, 93

Quicksand or Concrete, 108

R

Railroad Tracks, Not Tightrope, 122

Rear Foot Is the Rudder of a Ship, 121

Regrip at the Top, 251

Relate, Don't One-Up, 377

Respect the Timeline, 384

Responsibility, 290

Rest in the Nest, 195

Resting at the Free-Throw Line, 85

Rib Cage to Pelvis, 41

Rib Down, Press Down, 53

Rising Tide Lifts All Boats, A, 342

Rocket Fuel Stages, 176

Roll to Elbow, 202

Rower's Happy Hour, 218

Rowing Sequence, 214–215

Rubber Ball Bounce, 174

S

Same, Better, or Worse, 373

Same Message, Fewer Words, 374

Saw Don't Chop, 209

Say No to the Bow, 260

Scoop, The, 153

Screw Your Feet into the Floor, 13

See Your Big Toe, 15

Seesaw, 117

Set an Intent and Purpose, 275

Sharpen Your Axe, 348

Show Me How Fat You Are, 235

Show Me the Armpits, 31

Show Me Your Shirt, 18

Silverback Stance, 184

Sleep Is the Greatest Legal Performance-Enhancing Drug, 338

Slow Down, 316

Smaller the Steps, the Longer the Journey, The, 331

Snatch, The, 127

Snatch Balance & Drop Snatch, 136

Sometimes It's Okay to Spill a Little Tea, 317

Space Is Weakness, 94

Spend Less Time Scrollin' and More Time Pullin', 301

Spin the Earth, 210

Spine Above Shoulder Blades, 43

Split Jerk, 103

Split Jerk Receiving Position, 106

Split Jerk Setup & Landing, 107

Split Jerk Trailing Foot Position, 120

Spread the Towel, 21

Squat Is Essential to Your Well-Being, The, 19

Squat the Bar with Your Hands, 23

Squatting→Sitting on the Toilet, 11

Squeeze Oranges, 95

Stair Steps, 213

Stance, Grip, Positioning, 252

Stand at Attention, 68

Stand Like a Superhero, 96

Standing Broad Jump, 44

Start Position, 128

Stay in the Phone Booth, 72

Straight Through the Roof!, 171

Strength Training Basics, 389

Strength Triangle, The, 393

Stress/Growth Continuum, 329

Strict Muscle-Up, 54

Strong People Are Harder to Kill, 310

Swing, Pull, Punch, 197

Synergists, Not Opposites, 336

T

Take the Elevator, Not the Stairs, 173

Tall Jerk, 104

Tap, Shoot, Reload, 73

Technical Lingo < Understanding, 359

Teeth Brushing and Training, 330

Think Box & Play Box, 276

Three Best Friends, The, 79

Thumb to Bum, 198

Thumbs Touch Side of Thighs, 254

Thumbs Trace Your Chest, 55

Tight Core Helps You Lift More, A, 231

Tighter = Lighter, in Olympic lifting, 175

Tighter = Lighter, when bracing, 237

To Be a Great Teacher, You Must Also Be a Great Student, 361

Toes & Traps, 154

Toes Are a Paintbrush, 42

Towel Between the Feet, 57

Training = Move the Dirt, 324

Trap Door, 162

Treat 135# Like Your Max, 277

Tripod, 38

Try a Criticism Sandwich, 368

Tuck the Butt, 65

Two Buttons, 188

U–V

Uncooked Spaghetti, Not Cooked Spaghetti, 66

Uniforms Are Key, 380

Use Your Ears, 364

Use Your Thumb as a Sight, 201

Use Your Thumbs, 253

Voice Inside Your Head, The, 332

W

We Don't Stop Moving Because We Grow Old, 309

Wet Towel Snap to the Rear, 193

What Makes a Good Coach?, 350

When Animals Surrender They Go Lying on Their Back, 294

When Fisherman Can't Go to Sea, They Mend Their Nets, 339

When the Arms Bend, the Power Ends, 155

When Training Gets Tough, 304

When Weaknesses Improve, Overall Fitness Increases, 392

Where Is Your Focus, 305

Work Hard & Be Nice to People, 292

Y

Yelling Is a Weakness, 378

You Bully the Bar, 278

You Can't Push a Wall Over if You Never Touch It, 328

You Must Be Aggressive, 306

Your Lift Starts Here, 279